AF449215

Conservation Surgery and Radiation Therapy in the Treatment of Operable Breast Cancer

Frontiers of Radiation Therapy and Oncology

Vol. 17

Editor
Jerome M. Vaeth, San Francisco, Calif.

Associate Editors
Jerold P. Green, Alan F. Schröder, Simeon T. Cantril and
Mary Louise Meurk

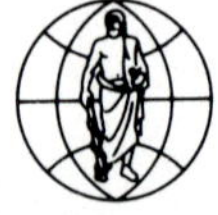

S. Karger · Basel · München · Paris · London · New York · Sydney

17th Annual San Francisco Cancer Symposium, San Francisco, Calif.
February 27–28, 1982

Conservation Surgery and Radiation Therapy in the Treatment of Operable Breast Cancer

Editor
Jerome M. Vaeth, San Francisco, Calif.

17 figures and 33 tables, 1983

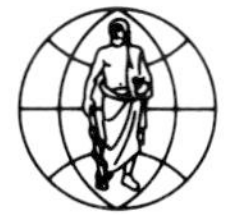

S. Karger · Basel · München · Paris · London · New York · Sydney

Frontiers of Radiation Therapy and Oncology

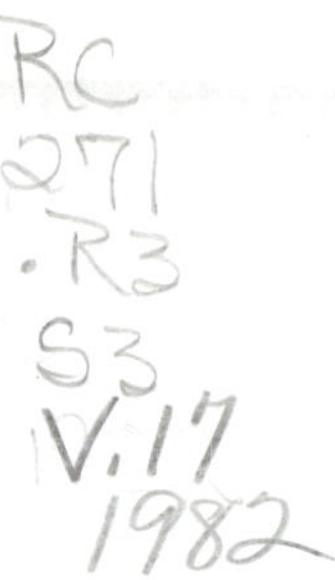

Drug Dosage

The authors and the publisher have exerted every effort to ensure that drug selection and dosage set forth in this text are in accord with current recommendations and practice at the time of publication. However, in view of ongoing research, changes in government regulations, and the constant flow of information relating to drug therapy and drug reactions, the reader is urged to check the package insert for each drug for any change in indications and dosage and for added warnings and precautions. This is particularly important when the recommended agent is a new and/or infrequently employed drug.

Contents

Foreword

For decades, arising from Halsted's classic work, the radical mastectomy and later the modified radical mastectomy have dominated the management of breast cancer. Running parallel to the surgical dominance was a growing experience in the application of radiation therapy, both adjunctive and definitive, in the treatment of early carcinoma of the breast. Only in recent years has the concept of tylectomy (lumpectomy or conservation surgery) and radiation therapy challenged the modified radical mastectomy as an alternative treatment method for women who view breast preservation as an important aspect of the management of this disease.

On February 27–28, 1982, the 17th Annual San Francisco Cancer Symposium entitled 'Conservation Surgery and Radiation Therapy in the Treatment of Breast Cancer' addressed the issues related to this acceptable and perhaps preferable conservative approach. The faculty conducting the symposium represented the dominant institutions of the world knowledgeable in the subject. We hope the information generated by the Symposium will further benefit the thousands of women who will develop breast cancer, and temper some of the surgical bias and misinformation that has existed for decades and still today in the management of this common and deadly disease.

The symposium was generously supported by the California Division of the American Cancer Society, Varian Associates, Adria Laboratories, Alpha Omega Services, Inc., Mead Johnson, Ross Laboratories, Siemens Corporation, E. R. Squibb and Sons, Inc., and Stuart Pharmaceuticals.

Jerome M. Vaeth, San Francisco, Calif.

Front. Radiat. Ther. Onc., vol. 17, pp. 1–10 (Karger, Basel 1983)

Historical Aspects of Tylectomy and Radiation Therapy in the Treatment of Cancer of the Breast

Jerome M. Vaeth

Department of Radiation Therapy, St. Mary's Hospital and Medical Center,
San Francisco, Calif., USA

Were it not for the pioneering work of earlier dedicated radiation therapists, women today might still not be offered an alternative to the disfiguring mastectomy. The concept that a woman might be cured of her cancer of the breast by conservation surgery (preserving the majority of the breast) and the judicious application of ionizing radiations is based on this fundamental premise:

Ionizing radiations can sterilize adenocarcinoma of the breast at its primary site as well as in the breast's regional lymphatics.

For those of us who have irradiated extensive cancers of the breast and bulky nodal metastases and observed regression and disappearance of malignant tumors, this premise is not difficult to accept. Yet for decades, the majority of medical and surgical specialists, including many a radiation therapist, have perpetuated the myth that cancer of the breast is radiation resistant, that only surgery removing the cancer and the invaded organ offered a chance of cure, and further that if the cancer had spread beyond the breast, the woman was incurable.

Although *Roentgen* is credited by most to have discovered x-rays in November 1895, a considerable amount of research in vacuum tubes preceded *Roentgen's* announcement. In 1859 *Plücker* [55] of Germany reported on a fluorescence produced on the inner wall of a Geissler low-vacuum tube by a ray labeled a cathode ray by *Hittorf* [29] in 1869. Further research in vacuum tubes was advanced when *Crookes* [12] in 1875, using high vacuum tubes, duplicated *Hittorf's* experiments revealing that solid materials placed in the cathode ray would cast a shadow on the inner glass wall of the tube – the first x-ray image. *Jackson* [30], in 1894, improving on the design of *Crookes's* tubes, pioneered the use of the angled platinum anodes, studied chemicals which would give off 'phosphorescence', and devised the x-ray tube that would become a standard design for years to come. *Lenard* [41], working with his mentor, *Heinrich Hertz*, in Germany, and expanding on *Hertz's* earlier vacuum tube research, reported in September 1895, that cathode rays would excite barium cyanide crystals to fluorescence even when his hand was placed between *Crookes's* tube and the barium cyanide crystals. In June, 1895, *Wiedmann* [64] discovered that some of the rays produced by the Crookes tube were not magnetically deflected.

Wilhelm Roentgen, while duplicating some of *Lenard's* earlier experiments, expanded on *Lenard's* findings and covered *Crookes's* tube with black paper to exclude ultraviolet radiations as a source of fluorescence. He darkened the room, then holding a box of loosely arranged barium platinum cyanide crystals with his hand under the box and over *Crookes's* tube, observed to his amazement the bones of his hand duplicated in the fluorescent crystals – this on November 5, 1895. The following day, he submitted a written report of his findings. This report was published 2 days later on November 8, 1895 [58]. *Roentgen* named these rays x-rays.

But 60 days after *Roentgen's* epic announcement on January 29, 1896, an ambitious young 2nd-year medical student, *Emil H. Grubbe,* irradiated the first cancer patient in his Chicago vacuum tube factory. The patient, Mrs. Rose Lee, suffered from an extensive carcinoma of the left breast and was referred by *R. Ludlam,* one of *Grubbe's* medical school professors [25]. This physician had observed *Grubbe's* radiation dermatitis of the hand at the medical school and proposed that perhaps these very active rays might destroy malignant tissue as well as normal tissue. *Grubbe,* undoubtedly the world's first radiation therapist, wisely protected the woman's normal tissues from the x-rays by shielding them with lead foil from a Chinese tea box. Later *Grubbe* graduated from Hahnemann Medical College and continued to practice radiation therapy, becoming professor of roentgenology at that school, probably the world's first professor of roentgenology (fig. 1).

In 1897 *Gocht* [24] reported the successful results of roentgen therapy of 2 patients with breast cancer. These were epic times in the management of breast cancer. Just 2 years before *Grubbe's* achievement in 1894, *Halsted* [28] and *Meyer* made the radical mastectomy the gold standard against which all procedures would be measured and judged.

In 1901, the year following *Marie and Pierre Curie's* [13] isolation of radium from pitchblende, a patient with a skin disorder was treated with

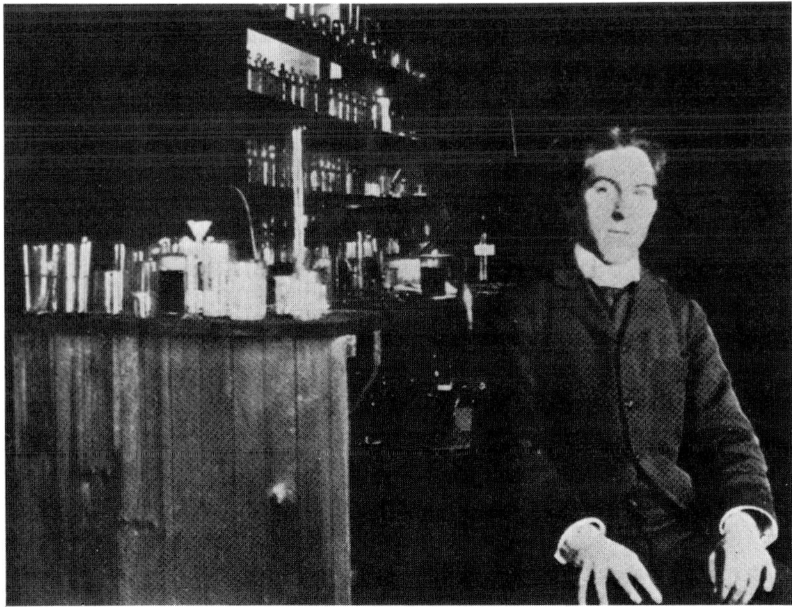

Fig. 1. E. H. Grubbe, pioneer radiation therapist, in his Chicago laboratory.

radium. It was inevitable that cancer of the breast would be treated by radium applications. Indeed, in 1914, *Rauschoff* [56] reported the impressive result he achieved in irradiating a woman with an over 5-cm diameter lesion of the upper outer quadrant but with no palpable axillary lymphadenopathy. The mass was not excised. 8 years after three separate 24-hour applications of 100 mg radium, his patient was alive, well and free of recurrence with the breast intact.

Janeway [31] in 1917 reported on the interstitial irradiation of operable breast cancer in lieu of mastectomy and stated, 'The use of radium can be offered to those patients who dread and refuse operation and it should also be useful in cases where the wisdom of using the knife is doubtful'.

Credit for the development and practice of tylectomy and radiation therapy in a systematic fashion undoubtedly belongs to *Geoffrey Keynes*. In 1924 at St. Bartholomew's Hospital, *Keynes* began the routine practice of tylectomy followed by radium application to the entire breast and nodal drainage in operable carcinoma (fig. 2). In following papers in 1929 [36] and 1937 [37], *Keynes* stressed the importance of tumor removal followed by

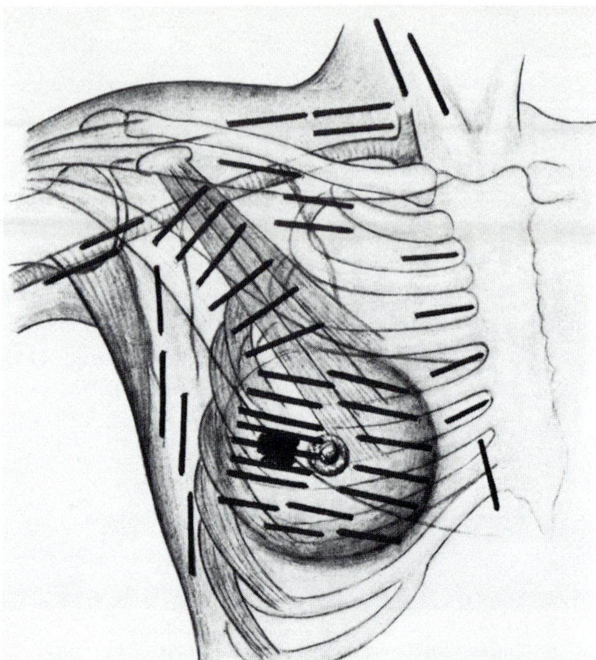

Fig. 2. Technique of radium implantation following tylectomy as practiced by *Keynes* in 1924. Note that the entire breast, including tylectomy site, chest wall, and nodal drainage sites, is irradiated.

interstitial radium to the breast and regional nodes and 'not needling alone, except in selected cases', as well as the excellent local/regional control of the disease and cosmetic appearance of the intact breast. Sir *Stanford Cade* [10], a colleague of *Keynes,* also was an early advocate of this philosophy and technique. In his classic textbook, *Malignant Disease and Its Treatment by Radium,* he describes in detail the selection of patients, the technique of the interstitial radium treatment and his results. Photographs showing his excellent cosmetic results rival those of the best achieved by modern-day radiation therapists.

Perhaps because of the complexities of delivering ionizing radiations with primitive x-ray generators and the lack of reproducible dose, curie-therapy was to be the dominant radiotherapeutic modality in the treatment of breast cancer in the twenties. Only in 1928 was the roentgen accepted as the unit of dose, the determination based on the ionization of gases. The combined use of x-rays and radium in large numbers of breast cancer patients (27 cases) treated between 1902 and 1928, was reported by *Pfahler* [54] in 1938 and *Maisin* in 1939 [45].

Much information, particularly histological evidence of the effects of radiations on breast cancer, was gained by preoperative radiation series in the 1920s and 1930s. This information was to serve a useful purpose as substantiating the validity of the concept of tumor control by tylectomy and radiation therapy. In 1921 *Haendly* [27] and 2 years later *DeBacker and Derom* [14] reported on the histology of preoperatively irradiated breast cancer. In subsequent years an entire literature was developed on this subject by investigators: *Neuman* et al. [50] (1924), *Laborde* [39] (1925), *Lee and Herendeen* [40] (1925), *Berven* [6] (1929), *Adair* [1] (1936), Pfahler [54] (1938), [53] (1932). Often these results were conflicting, but we must remember that equipment was primitive, and, in general, the doses of radiations administered were low by today's standards. Nevertheless, the evidence was clear that ionizing radiations could influence cancer of the breast.

It was not until *Maurice Lenz's* well documented work from 1933 through 1937 (published in 1936 [42] and 1947 [43]) described the relationship that exists between the tumor size, the dose of radiations administered and tumor sterilization. Since *Lenz's* reports, an impressive array of preoperative irradiation series has evolved which supported *Lenz's* observations and added further proof of the ability of ionizing radiations to sterilize breast cancer [5, 7, 8, 11, 15, 16, 20–23, 32, 35, 38, 44, 57, 59–63, 65].

Despite the growing encyclopedia of information on the potential of radiation therapy in the management of early breast cancer, the radical mastectomy had assumed almost divine status and became the gold standard by which the worth of all procedures was judged. Lest we forget, there were many well-trained surgeons but few trained radiation therapists during this era.

The first substantial radiation therapy challenge to the radical mastectomy was issued by *McWhirter* [47] in 1949 when he published his results in the use of the simple mastectomy with postoperative medium-voltage x-ray therapy as a routine procedure in breast cancer treatment. He substantiated that the number of local recurrences could be minimized and axillary lymph node metastases could be controlled by radiation therapy. Further, the survival figures closely approximated those of the radical mastectomy. This concept was confirmed by *Kaae and Johansen* comparing the results in operable patients with an extended radical mastectomy group and reported in 1959 [33] and 1965 [34]. This report was further substantiated by *Brinkley and Haybittle's* [9] work at Cambridge reported in 1968 and *Maisin* et al. [46] in 1973. If, indeed, we compared the results of simple mastectomy and radiation therapy in terms of 5- and 10-year recurrence-free survival with the results of the radical mastectomy, we could justify the simple mastectomy/radiation therapy technique as a routine method of treatment. It follows that if breast preservation is an important goal in the treatment of early disease, the results of simple mastectomy/radiation therapy can be duplicated by conservation surgery (tylectomy) and radiation therapy.

Running parallel to the experience gained in preradical mastectomy radiation therapy and simple mastectomy with postoperative radiation therapy was that of definitive radiation therapy with or without primary tumor removal. Tylectomy and Curie therapy as practiced and reported by *Keynes* [36] (1929) and *Cade* [11] (1929) preceded by 10 years the first published tylectomy/roentgentherapy reports.

The early literature of tylectomy/radiation therapy is sparse. A cluster of investigators stand out in these earlier years as the pioneers of lumpectomy and x-ray therapy of early breast cancers – *Baclesse* [2, 4], *Evans and Leucutia* [18], *Pendergrass and Hodes* [51]. In 1939, a report by *Maisin* et al. [46] also substantiated *Baclesse's* observations. Meanwhile, in Helsinki, *Mustakallio* [49] was methodically documenting 702 cases treated in this fashion from 1937. His report in 1954 [49] echoed *Baclesse's* and *Maisin's* conclusions with even more substantial numbers. *DeWinter* [17] in 1961 reported his successful experience in this technique. In 1965 *Fletcher and Montague* [19] reported their experience at M.D. Anderson Hospital in both early and advanced cases. They established the basic premise that cancer of the breast can be sterilized both at its primary site and in its regional lymphatic drainage sites by ionizing radiations.

Guttman [26] from New York in 1962 wrote of a remarkable experience. She, by irradiating the 'rejects' of Haagenson's radical mastectomy (rejected by virtue of a positive biopsy of the internal mammary and/or high axillary lymph nodes), reported excellent local regional control and long-term survival. Treatment was directed to the breast including the excision biopsy site as well as the chest wall and the nodal draining regions. *Peters* [52] from Toronto accumulated a large series of cases treated by wedge resection and radiation therapy and reported in 1967.

At this time (50s, 60s and 70s), several other events, medical and nonmedical, occurred which were to influence the methods of management of this disease. In the surgical world growing skepticism of the value of the radical mastectomy versus the morbidity drove surgeons to a less radical procedure, the modified radical mastectomy. Women of the world accustomed to the freedom both in body and spirit bred from World War II began to demand a voice in decision making on medical matters related to their bodies. For many, the radical mastectomy, even the modified radical mastectomy, was an operative procedure to be entered into only after explanations of its benefits but also of alternatives to this procedure. Right or wrong, some states felt a necessity to enact legislation to insure a woman of her medical rights to proper information in the treatment of cancer of the breast (Massachusetts, California).

Over half a century ago, Sir *Geoffrey Keynes* pointed the way. In the 1970s there are more than 25 reports, well documented and with hundreds of cases followed to observe not only recurrence-free survival, but as well the side effects of treatment and cosmetic results. These reports continue to accumulate arising from highly regarded cancer centers of the world. Several of these reports are published in this text. Surely such reports should not go unnoticed.

Only a few hundred patients entered into earlier modified radical mastectomy series eased our surgical colleagues into accepting this less mutilating procedure for their patients. How many thousands of cured and nonmaimed patients must the radiation therapists of the world accumulate before tylectomy and radiation therapy takes its place as an acceptable method of treatment of early carcinoma of the breast?

References

1 Adair, F. E.: The effect of preoperative irradiation in primary operable cancer of the breast. Am. J. Roentg. *35:* 359–370 (1936).
2 Baclesse, F.; Gricouroff, G.; Tailhefer, A.: Essai de rœntgenthérapie du cancer du sein suivie d'opération large. Résultats histologiques. Bull. Cancer *28:* 729–743 (1939).
3 Baclesse, F.: La rœntgenthérapie seule employée dans le traitement des cancers du sein, opérables et inopérables. J. Radiol. Electrol. *30:* 323 (1949).
4 Baclesse, F.: Roentgentherapy as the sole method of treatment of cancer of the breast. Am. J. Roentg. *62:* 311–319 (1949).
5 Baclesse, F.: A method of preoperative roentgentherapy by high doses followed by radical operation for carcinoma of the breast (showing survivals up to 10 years). J. Fac. Radiol. *6:* 145–163 (1955).
6 Berven, E.: The technique at Radiumhemmet in the treatment of tumours except cancer uteri. Acta Radiol. *10:* 3–48 (1929).

7   Berven, E.: Die Strahlenbehandlung des Mammakarzinoms. Fortschr. Geb. Röntg-
      Strahl. *75:* 10–25 (1951).
8   Bouchard, J.: Advanced cancer of the breast treated primarily with irradiation.
      Radiology *84:* 823–841 (1965).
9   Brinkley, D.; Haybittle, J.L.: A 15-year follow-up study of patients treated for
      carcinoma of the breast. Br. J. Radiol. *41:* 215–221 (1968).
10   Cade, S.: Malignant disease and its treatment by radium (Williams & Wilkins, Baltimore
      1940).
11   Cade, S.: Treatment and results in cancer of the breast. Am. J. Roentg. *62:* 326–327
      (1949).
12   Crookes, W.: Quoted by Grubbe, E.H.: Priority in the therapeutic use of x-rays.
      Radiology *21:* 156–162 (1933).
13   Curie, P.; Curie, M.: Sur une substance nouvelle radioactive, contenue dans la
      pechblende. C. r. hebd. Acad. Sci., Paris *127:* 175 (1898).
14   DeBacker, P.; Derom, F.: Contribution à l'étude des formes de regression de tumeurs
      malignes sous l'action de l'irradiation. Bull. Cancer *12:* 635–663 (1923).
15   Delarue, N.; Ash, C.; Peters, V.; Fielder, R.: Preoperative irradiation in management
      of locally advanced breast cancer. Archs. Surg., Chicago *91:* 136–154 (1965).
16   de Schoyver, A.: The Stockholm breast cancer trial: preliminary report of a randomized
      study concerning the value of preoperative or postoperative radiotherapy in operable
      disease. Int. J. Radiol. Oncol. Biol. Physics *1:* 601–609 (1976).
17   DeWinter, J.G.: Early breast cancer treated by biopsy excision and radiotherapy: a
      preliminary report; in Rajewsky, 9th Int. Congr. Radiol., München 1959, vol.1,
      pp.781–782 (Thieme, Stuttgart 1961).
18   Evans, W.A.; Leucutia, T.: Deep roentgen ray therapy of mammary carcinoma. Am. J.
      Roentg. *42:* 866–881 (1939).
19   Fletcher, G.H.; Montague, E.D.: Radical irradiation of advanced breast cancer. Am. J.
      Roentg. *93:* 573 (1965).
20   Fletcher, G.H.: The advantages of preoperative irradiation. J. Am. med. Ass. *200:*
      140–141 (1967).
21   Fletcher, G.H.; Montague, E.D.; White, E.C.: Radiation therapy in the primary
      management of breast cancer. Prog. clin. Cancer *4:* 242–256 (1970).
22   Fletcher, G.H.: Local results of irradiation in the management of localized breast
      cancer. Cancer *29:* 545–551 (1972).
23   Fletcher, G.H.: Textbook of radiotherapy: 2nd ed., pp.457–493 (Lea & Febiger,
      Philadelphia, 1973).
24   Gocht, H.: Therapeutische Verwendungen der Röntgenstrahlen. Fortschr. Geb. Röntg-
      Strahl. *1:* 14–22 (1897).
25   Grubbe, E.H.: X-ray treatment, its origin, birth and early history (Bruce, 1949).
26   Guttman, R.J.: Survival and results after 2 million volt irradiation in the treatment of
      primary operable carcinoma of the breast with proved positive internal mammary and/or
      highest axillary nodes. Cancer *15:* 383–386 (1962).
27   Haendly, P.: Pathologisch-anatomische Ergebnisse der Strahlenbehandlung, Strahlen-
      therapie *12:* 1–87 (1921).
28   Halsted, W.S.: The result of operations for cure of the cancer of the breast performed at
      the Johns Hopkins Hospital. Ann. Surg. *20:* 497–555 (1894).
29   Hittorf, J.: Ann. Poggendorf *136* (1869).

30 Jackson, H.: Quoted by Grubbe, E.H., Priority in the therapeutic use of x-rays. Radiology *21:* 156–162 (1933).

31 Janeway, H.H.: Radium therapy in cancer at Memorial Hospital, N.Y., pp.184–190 (Hober, 1917).

32 Kaae, S.: The value of preoperative irradiation in operable breast cancer. Acta radiol. *37:* 576–586 (1952).

33 Kaae, S.; Johansen, H.: Breast cancer: comparison of results of simple mastectomy with post-operative roentgen irradiation by McWhirter method with those of extended radical mastectomy. Acta radiol. *188:* 155–161 (1959).

34 Kaae, S.; Johansen, H.: Simple mastectomy plus post-operative irradiation by the method of McWhirter for mammary carcinoma. Prog. clin. Cancer *1:* 453–461 (1965).

35 Kahr, E.; Schreyer, H.: Zur Frage der präoperativen Bestrahlung des Mammakarzinoms im Stadium I und IIa. Strahlentherapie *130:* 481–488 (1966).

36 Keynes, G.: The treatment of primary carcinoma of the breast with radium. Acta radiol. *10:* 393–402 (1929).

37 Keynes, G.: Conservative treatment of cancer of the breast. Br. med. J. *ii:* 643–647 (1937).

38 Kohler, A.: 10 Jahre präoperative Bestrahlung des Mamma-Carcinoms, Strahlentherapie *88:* 150–163 (1952).

39 Laborde, S.: La curiethérapie des cancers, pp.245–248 (Masson, Paris 1925).

40 Lee, B.J.; Herendeen, R.E.: An evaluation of pre-operative and post-operative radiation in the treatment of mammary carcinomas. Ann. Surg. *82:* 404–412 (1925).

41 Lenard, P.: Quoted by Grubbe, E.H.: Priority in the therapeutic use of x-rays. Radiology *21:* 156–162 (1933).

42 Lenz, M.: Tumor dosage and results in roentgen therapy of cancer of the breast. Am. J. Roentg. *56:* 67–74 (1936).

43 Lenz, M.: Tissue dosage in roentgen therapy of mammary cancer. Acta radiol. *28:* 583–592 (1947).

44 Lindgren, M.; Borgström, S.; Landberg, T.: Pre-operative radiotherapy in operable breast cancer; in: Prognostic factors in breast cancer. Proc. 1st Tenovus Symposium 1967, pp.103–107 Livingstone, Edinburgh 1968).

45 Maisin, J.; Estas, P.; Line, D.: Le traitement du cancer du sein par le radium et les rayons x. Bull. Cancer *29:* 712–728 (1939).

46 Maisin, H.E.; Braeker, G.; Wanbersie, A.; Keusfeis, J.. Résultats comparés des traitements radiologiques et radio-chirurgicaux des cancers du sein de stades I et II. Radiol. clin. biol. *42:* 177–190 (1973).

47 McWhirter, R.: Carcinoma of the breast. Am. J. Roentg. *62:* 335–340 (1949).

48 Muntean, E.: Zur präoperativen Röntgenbestrahlung des Mamma-Karzinoms. Fortschr. Geb. RöntgStrahl. *104:* 546–553.

49 Mustakallio, S.: Treatment of breast cancer by tumour extirpation and roentgentherapy instead of radical operation. J. Fac. Radiol. *6:* 23–26 (1954).

50 Neuman; Stuys, F.; Coryn: Technique radiochirurgicale des cancers du sein. Archs. Electr. Med. *32:* 33–36 (1924).

51 Pendergrass, E.P.; Hodes, P.J.: Further observations on carcinoma of the breast. Am. J. Roentg. *42:* 393–402 (1939).

52 Peters, M.V.. Wedge reoection and irradiation, an effective treatment in early breast cancer. J. Am. med. Ass. *200:* 144 (1967).

53 Pfahler, G.E.: Results of radiation therapy in 1022 private cases of carcinoma of the breast from 1902 to 1928 (including 127 cases in which radium and roentgen rays were combined). Am. J. Roentg. *27:* 497–508 (1932).

54 Pfahler, G.E.: The treatment of carcinoma of the breast. Am. J. Roentg. *39:* 1–18 (1938).

55 Plücker, J.: Quoted by Grubbe, E.H.: Priority in the therapeutic use of x-rays. Radiology *21:* 156–162 (1933).

56 Rauschoff, J.L.: Inoperable carcinoma of the breast clinically cured by radium. Lancet-Clin. *112:* 618 (1914).

57 Richards, G.E.: Mammary cancer. The place of surgery and of radiotherapy in its management. I. A study of some of the factors which determine success or failure in treatment. Br. J. Radiol. *21:* 109–127 (1948).

58 Roentgen, W.G.: Über eine neue Art von Strahlen. Sber. phys.-med. Ges. Würzb. *30:* 132–141 (1895).

59 Schinz, H.R.; Botsztejn, C.: Der Brustkrebs in Zürich. Oncology *1:* 91–109 (1948).

60 Vaeth, J.M.; Clark, J.C.; Green, J.P.; Schroeder, A.F.; Lowy, R.O.: Radiotherapeutic management of locally advanced carcinoma of the breast. Cancer *30:* 107–112 (1972).

61 Vaeth, J.M.: Inflammatory cancer of the breast, Encyclopedia of medical radiology, vol. XIX 2 (Springer, Berlin 1980).

62 Wallgarn, A.; Arner, O.; Bergström, J.; Blomstedt, B.; Granberg, P.O.; Karnström, L.; Räf, L.; Silferswärd, C.: The value of preoperative radiotherapy in operable mammary carcinoma. Int. J. Radiol. Oncol. Biol. Phys. *6:* 287–290 (1980).

63 Widow, W.; Marx, G.; Peck, U.: Die Behandlung des operablen Brustdrüsenkrebses; in: Gummel, Widow, Symposium über den Brustdrüsenkrebs, 1973, pp. 71–83.

64 Wiedmann, M.: Z. Elektrochem. *7* (1895); quoted by Grubbe, E.H.: X-ray treatment, its origin, birth and early history (Bruce, 1949).

65 Zuppinger, A.: Die präbioptische Bestrahlung beim Mammakarzinom; in Neue Aspekte der Krebsbekämpfung, pp. 101–107 (Thieme, Stuttgart 1979).

Dr. Jerome M. Vaeth, Department of Radiation Therapy, St. Mary's Hospital and Medical Center, Hayes and Stanyan Street, San Francisco, CA 94117 (USA)

Front. Radiat. Ther. Onc., vol. 17, pp. 11–15 (Karger, Basel 1983)

'High Risk' Women:
Breast Cancer Concerns and Health Practices[1]

Patricia T. Kelly

Stanton and Corinne Sobel Genetic Counseling Service, Department of Medicine, Mount Zion Hospital and Medical Center, San Francisco, Calif., USA

Introduction

I am a medical geneticist who specializes in giving women information about their breast cancer risk. Most of the women I see have a family history of breast cancer. Generally, these women believe they are at very high risk of breast cancer. Their concern about risk is sometimes warranted and sometimes not. A family history of breast cancer can increase a woman's risk considerably [1]. In fact, it used to be thought that all women who had a close relative with breast cancer had a risk two to four times greater than that of women who had no such family history [2].

Anderson of the M. D. Anderson Hospital and Tumor Institute has shown that not all women who have a family history of breast cancer are at the same high risk. Instead, even women with similar appearing family histories can have very different risks. He has found that women whose relatives had premenopausal, bilateral breast cancer are generally at higher risk than are those whose relatives had postmenopausal, unilateral disease [3].

In my practice, I have found that it is not enough to present risk information to patients in a clear fashion. Women with a family history of breast cancer also need help in integrating the risk information into their own lives and value systems [4]. Without this help, I find that the patients I see do not know how to make use of the information they receive.

[1] This work was supported in part by the Research Support Program of the Mount Zion Hospital and Medical Center, San Francisco, and by grant No. CA 09348 from the National Institute of Health.

I will report on some of the reactions of women who have a family history of breast cancer, particularly those reactions that can impede information transfer or inhibit the implementation of reasonable breast health practices.

Emotional Aspects

The reader may have noticed that the title of this paper has high risk in quotes. The quotes are to signify that women who have a family history of breast cancer are not all at high risk; however, most believe that they are. Often patients tell me that they are virtually certain to get breast cancer, or that their risk is 150%.

I once did a tally of 168 consecutive patients who had a family history of breast cancer. Of these, 51% thought their risks were higher than they actually were, 22% thought they were lower, and 27% thought they were about what they actually were. But nearly all thought of themselves as high risk women.

Fear

It is not surprising that the most common reaction to breast cancer in a family member is fear. Women fear: the disfigurement they think is always associated with breast cancer, the threat to their lives, and they fear the disruption to their own and their families' lives if they should get breast cancer.

As one woman said:

'It would be unpleasant to loose a breast, but dying the horrible death my mother died ... I'll never forget it. The three children knew, everyone knew there was a waiting period until she died. The operation was very painful and the scar was hideous. It was difficult to simulate normal appearance. Then she found out she had one year to live. She was in pain all the time. She hated putting her family through it. The end is horrible. You get thin and your hair falls out. The cost was horrible. My father himself paid over $ 70,000 plus the insurance. I was going back and forth, but it was hard for my family to pay for my air fare. I couldn't stand to stay there and watch mother waste away. Mother hated for me to be there and wanted me there at the same time. Our family situation deteriorated. All of us children married people we wouldn't have otherwise. We all got away from home in the only acceptable way.'

The fear of cancer is always present in some women even years after their relative died of breast cancer. For example, one woman said:

'When my sister and I get sick we worry. I don't think I have cancer, but if I have even a cold there's a taste of anxiety underneath.'

Some patients are subject to a sudden and intense wave of fear that is almost incapacitating. One woman became convinced she had breast cancer because her doctor looked grave during her routine visit and did not engage in his customary small talk with her. She was terrified. Fortunately, I knew her physician and was able to tell her the reason for his behavior – his wife had been suddenly hospitalized the day before.

Even women whose relatives had breast cancer and lived are terrified of this disease. They know only too well how the loss of a breast and the loss of arm function affected their mothers.

Here is how some daughters described the effect of their mother's mastectomy:

'It didn't seem like she felt well. She would just sit around. She had this large arm that seemed to be giving her more trouble than anything else.'

'Emotionally, I don't think she ever got over it. She didn't adjust to her breast being gone. She needed compassion from my stepfather and he wasn't able to really give it to her and make her feel like she was a whole woman. Her breasts were one of her prides in life. She had a large bust as a young woman and she never really adjusted.'

'My mother almost passed out when she first saw her scar. It was really a blow. I'm a nurse, and I've seen this happen to a lot of women, so I was prepared for it. I had to put her head between her knees.'

Guilt

Guilt is another frequent reaction to breast cancer in the family. No matter how much attention women gave their affected relative, they feel it was not enough. Some, like the woman quoted earlier, went back and forth between their mother and a distant town. Some were so upset that they saw little of their affected cancer relative. Still others were present, but now feel they did not do enough or show enough sympathy:

'I must have known she had breast cancer when she had her breast removed. But they just used the word tumor. I asked her, and she said she didn't have breast cancer. But I must have known. I just can't remember!'

Some feel guilty about the way they behaved to their unaffected parent:

'I wasn't a nice girl. I acted out and I hated my father. I hated him for years. He never would tell me that she was going to die. He always acted like everything would be all right and I knew it wouldn't. I guess I hated him for his inability to not make things OK. He wasn't a Daddy.'

Some even feel they may be responsible for their relative's cancer:

'I've often wondered if my mother got cancer because she had four kids fourteen months apart. My grandmother used to say that if my mother hadn't had us kids so close together, she wouldn't have had cancer.'

Low Self-Esteem

As a result of low self-esteem, individuals may feel they are not intelligent enough to learn about effective breast health practices or the risk associated with breast cancer. Some feel that they are not worthy of information or of good medical care – or of taking up the doctor's time, even if they have a breast change or specific question about their breasts. One woman told me:

'I thought that I should do something concrete. I hate to take anybody's time, but I thought that maybe Dr. D. could look at it and tell me what he thinks about it. But then I've been here so many times when they have patients coming in because they are worried. They haven't asked me to come in extra, so I assume they aren't very worried about me. But you would hate to assume that and be wrong.'

Low self-esteem, fear and guilt can prevent high risk women (or women who are not at high risk, but who believe they are) from following even minimal breast health practices. Some of the women whose relatives had breast cancer are so emotionally upset about the disease that they cannot bring themselves to practice breast self-examination. Some are concerned that their emotional reactions to breast cancer might keep them from performing adequate breast examinations or might prevent them from rationally evaluating their findings. As one woman said:

'Any time I examine myself I have to face the question of whether there's something going on, and it's almost like I can't even ask myself that question. So I may examine myself, and I'll feel something, and I'll get anxious and say to myself, "Well, I know I'm anxious anyway, so how do I know what I feel?"'

Some of the women have such low self-esteem that they do not seek regular physician breast examinations. Some are so worried about breast cancer that they become concerned that ther physician will think they are hypochondriacs if they ask for several visits. Therefore, they space their visits to their gynecologist, allergist, internist and dermatologist and hope these physicians will offer to examine their breasts throughout the year. As you can imagine, many of these women do not practice regular breast self-examination, nor do they have regular breast examinations by a physician.

Conclusion

Clinicians have become increasingly aware of and attuned to the emotional and informational needs of breast cancer patients. I have tried to show that the relatives of breast cancer patients also have informational and emotional needs. Some of these needs are for: (1) information about their risk; (2) information about new treatments for breast cancer. They need to know that if they should get breast cancer they will not be subjected to the disfiguring treatments they remember their relatives had; and (3) counseling to help them make use of the information they receive, and to help them set up an effective health regimen for their breasts.

References

1   Anderson, D. E.: A genetic study of human breast cancer. J. natn. Cancer. Inst. *48:* 1029–1034 (1972).
2   Post, R. H.: Breast cancer, lactation, and genetics. Eugenics Quarterly *13:* 1–28 (1966).
3   Kelly, P. T.; Anderson, D. E.: Familial breast cancer: New data show lower risks for some sisters and daughters. Your Patient and Cancer, 25–32 (May 1981).
4   Kelly, P. T.: Counselling needs of women with a maternal history of breast cancer. Patient Counselling Health Education, *2:* 118–124 (1980).

P. T. Kelly, PhD, Director, Stanton and Corinne Sobel Genetic Counseling Service, Department of Medicine, Mount Zion Hospital and Medical Center, San Francisco, CA 94120 (USA)

Front. Radiat. Ther. Onc., vol. 17, pp. 16–22 (Karger, Basel 1983)

A Patient's Perspective of Conservation Surgery and Radiation Therapy

Aurore Vaeth

Mill Valley, Calif., USA

Lately, there has been much discussion and debate in both word and print, regarding breast cancer. The incidence, the etiology, the affected numbers, environmental concerns, chemicals, genetics, psychosocial aspects, and even the cancer personality. This particular symposium will delve into these matters in great detail. This paper, however, presents a very specific and personal viewpoint. It is a perspective of breast cancer, given by one who has seen the subject from a unique and very intimate vantage point.

'Grade I–II, infiltrating intraductal carcinoma of the left breast' – just a diagnosis on a pathology report. But when that diagnostic report bears your personal name, it is enough to turn your world into an earthquake eruption reaching ten-plus on the Richter Scale. From my nursing experience, I knew there were many medical problems as bad or far worse than cancer, and yet at 10.20 on a sunny February morning, my world became, at least for a period of time, as disheveled and uprooted as if I had been at the epicenter of the world's largest recorded earthquake.

Cancer is a six letter word, not one of those *bad* four letter words that make grandmothers and dowagers cringe, yet it can sound as repulsive and obscene as the worst of the four letter variety. Why is it, in this modern computerized scientific and sophisticated age, that the word 'cancer' still terrifies us and conjures up images of suffering and pain, images that existed back in the dark ages? Our anxieties regarding cancer seem to have no boundaries and we all react emotionally far out of proportion to the symptoms of the disease itself. It certainly is a life-threatening disease, but so is kidney disease, and we know that statistically, many more people die from cardiac disorders or cerebral vascular accidents.

So, for at least a measure of time, I found myself, not a clear-thinking, level-headed and sensible woman, but an emotional and distraught patient, devastated to learn the diagnosis of that simple little cyst-like tumor, removed only moments before in the emergency room.

I considered myself reasonably knowledgeable in the field of cancer. Not only had I worked as a surgical scrub nurse in the operating theater of a cancer hospital, but later in my nursing career, had been charge nurse on a pediatric oncology ward. Furthermore, my husband dealt with cancer patients on a daily basis and I had often helped abstract charts and search the medical literature for data for medical papers and talks on various aspects and types of cancer. And certainly, I was not worried about cancer personally. Longevity is a dominant trait in my family, particularly on my maternal side, and only one of those long-lived relatives had ever developed cancer – and he had been a heavy cigarette smoker for five decades and had died of pneumonia associated with cancer of the lung. Nor was there even a hint of cancer on my paternal side. In fact, there was nothing of note in my life that could be considered significant or tempting to the cancer fates, other than the fact that our first child was born when I was thirty.

I have always been a strong believer in the fact that God and/or fate, if you will, moves in an amazing way, and that there is, perhaps, always a reason for everything. A belief in God includes the comfortable feeling that there is order in the universe and in the overall design, every occurrence has a meaning, even if we do not always understand the implication at the time. Four months prior to my diagnosis of carcinoma of the breast, I had been forced to give a good deal of thought to what kind of treatment might be necessary, should such a diagnosis be made. At that time, I had discovered a lump in my right breast, and though mammography indicated nothing suspicious, the surgeon and I both agreed that it should be removed. A date was set for the week following my next menses. That gave me three weeks to research medical literature and ask a multitude of questions of medical friends. I already knew that I wanted a two-stage procedure, with the biopsy done first, and then if that lump should prove to be malignant, some time to make a rational decision on the proper mode of treatment. The surgeon was in accord with this approach, and it was agreed that should a frozen section show that the lump was malignant, he would also, at the same time, excise a sampling of the axillary lymph nodes which would be of obvious help in the staging of the disease, and would be an important aid in deciding the best course of treatment. Before I went to surgery for the biopsy, I knew that from my research and from my feelings about the matter, that should the lump be malignant, I would choose radiation therapy. I did not discuss this idea with the surgeon. Chemotherapy would be an important consideration only if the axillary nodes were positive or if there was evidence of metastases.

I must confess that I had a background in this, at that time, rather unconventional type of treatment. In 1957, I had nursed in Manchester, England, at the Christie Hospital and had frequently helped remove radium needles from tumor implants of breast patients. And later, in Paris, France, at the Fondation Curie, I observed that most cancer of the breast patients were treated by lumpectomy and radiation therapy, using equipment that was much less sophisticated than what is in use today. (I should add that as a Canadian trained RN, who had worked in the surgical theater of a well-known American cancer hospital, it was a definite shock to observe that in France, breast patients were not undergoing radical breast surgery. Remember that this was 1957 and it seemed like heresy!)

My biopsy was performed under general anesthesia and frozen sections done on the mass removed showed nothing malignant. Out of the recovery room and back in my room, my husband and I drank a bottle of champagne to celebrate – and from a combination of relief, medication, previous sleepless nights and the champagne, I slept the clock around in exhilarated exhaustion.

Six weeks later, on the return appointment to the surgeon's office for the official 'all clear', he discovered a small cyst-like mass on the upper outer quadrant, near the areola on the left breast – the opposite side. Since I was now diagnosed with that catch-all phrase of 'fibrocystic disease', and because a review of the mammography done two months previously showed nothing suspicious, he suggested we watch the lump for a month. The holidays passed by swiftly, followed by a trip to Hawaii. This lump was inclined to enlarge premenstrually and then decline in size. Nevertheless, it never disappeared and since a lump in the breast is an undesired lump in the breast, I wanted it removed. With the optimistic knowledge that 8 out of 10 breast masses are negative, I returned to the hospital to have this particular one excised. The champagne was again chilling and I had even arranged the emergency room appointment hour so my husband could take me out to lunch. As mentioned, it was a bright and sunny day.

There is something in the face of a friend bringing serious and/or bad news – embarrassment, sympathy, denial, helplessness – it was all there when the surgeon met my husband and me after the biopsy. He gave us the diagnosis but he had not really had to speak, for the news that this innocuous little swelling was really a mass of cells gone malignantly wild was evident by the look on his face. Images and thoughts run through your mind like a kaleidoscope gone wild – statistics, family reactions, whys and wherefores, the future of your three daughters, your own future – and yet it all seems unreal. Jerry took me home, all thoughts of a gala lunch and champagne gone.

The next few days were filled with activity and I was glad I had been forced to give this subject thought in those months before, because my research had been done and I knew the type of treatment I wanted to undergo. The laboratory work, including an SMA 12, as well as the usual routine items, chest X-rays and a bone scan all showed I was in good health with no obvious spread of disease.

When I firmly told my surgeon of my choice of treatment, he obviously thought I was foolhardy to embark on such a course of treatment, especially since he could give me all those glowing surgical statistics, essentially unchanged since Dr. Halsted performed the first radical mastectomy in 1894. He sincerely, I know, felt that surgery was the only answer to the problem and did indeed talk of reconstructive surgery in a very positive manner and urged me to have a consultation with a plastic surgeon. I opted for a consultation with a radiation oncologist instead, and my surgeon did accede to my wishes.

Five days after the initial biopsy, I returned to surgery where under general anesthesia, a wider excisional biopsy and a left axillary node dissection was performed. A very optimistic note was that neither the tissue in the wider excision nor any of the nodes removed from the axilla showed any sign of disease.

While still hospitalized – five days because of the rubber drains and dressings needed for the axillary dissection wound that oozed a great deal – a medical oncologist was called on consultation. After his examination, he agreed with the other physicians that chemotherapy was not warranted at this time, since no nodes had shown evidence of disease. He was pleasant and chatty, and as he was leaving, he noted that he could understand my vanity in refusing a mastectomy – but was I sure of my decision? My anger was explosive – vanity indeed – what about statistics? Medical literature shows that the 10-year follow-up survival studies done on those patients with this stage disease who had lumpectomy plus radiation therapy is identical to those who have undergone a mastectomy. Vanity indeed!

Postsurgery recovery was quick, once the drains were dispensed with, and my reach-to-recovery friend soon had me climbing with my fingertips up the door jams and washing windows. At least that was her idea of excellent postaxillary dissection exercise – the surgeon suggested that raising the main sail and pulling on the lines of the sailboat as more fun and equally good for me. I had to agree.

A month from the day of the biopsy, I started radiation therapy. During that month, I had been examined carefully, weighed, measured, had a complete physical exam, a CT scan of the chest and had a plaster contour made of my left chest wall. There was an entire team involved, including the radiation oncologists, medical physicists, dosimetrists, technicians, and nurses. Every aspect of the treatment was carefully planned and plotted by this team of experts for my particular case.

Treatments took place at first five times and later four times a week, for five weeks on the linear accelerator. Each treatment was exactly monitered and rarely took more than 20 minutes for the entire procedure, with much of that time taken up with the technician changing the treatment fields, since I was treated in several positions each day, tangential fields, to avoid any damage to lung tissue. The total treatment dose was 4,500 rads given on the linear accelerator and at the end of that treatment, a 'booster' dose was given the area where the tumor had originally been, by use of a cesuim unit. (This 'boost' is frequently given by introducing radioactive sources in the form of iridium seeds to the tumor site and is known as brachytherapy.)

One item of interest – no one told me to ignore my mother's sage advice about wearing ones best slip and bra when going to the doctors and I quickly learned that those indelible markings, used to reproduce the treatment field accurately, are only indelible on one's lingery, and that it was best to wear items that you did not mind seeing colored in such a fashion!

There were very few side effects and those were of little consequence. I drove myself into the city each day for treatment. Unlike the side effects experienced when many other parts of the body are treated by X-ray therapy, those produced by radiation of the breast are minimal – a slight cough, a mild esophagitis, and loss of hair under the left arm. The skin that was treated became less soft, was itchy, and a redness developed similar to a severe sunburn. Except for some degree of fatigue, I felt very well throughout treatment and continued all household and social activities, including the shopping and cooking for our three teenagers and their host of hungry friends – and hauling water, for those were the dry days of the great Marin drought. Of course, there was no nausea and no vomiting associated with treatment of breast cancer since the intestinal tract is not being irradiated, nor is there any loss of hair from the head, if no chemotherapeutic agents are used.

Important as they are for many patients undergoing treatment for cancer, the visualization techniques as described by the Drs. Simonton were of little or no value to me personally. I was never able to conjure up any appropriate images of my cancer, let alone see it in the form of, for example, a large chunk of raw meat being consumed by the X-rays which take the shape of a wonderfully large and fierce dog. I preferred to concentrate on the idea that there were *no* wild and uncontrollable things of any sort within my body and that my natural defenses were functioning just fine in cooperation with the treatment being received.

However, I do think it is important to mention that the love and support that I received, not only from my family and friends, but also from the medical personnel played no small part in my feelings of wellness.

Today, five years and two weeks later, I continue to feel well and am in excellent health. I see my doctors, both surgeon and radiation oncologist, every six months and have mammography annually. There was a time when the capriciousness of the disease dominated my thinking and at some time during every day, I would develop that clutch of fear, that grim reality of the fact that I had been treated for cancer. Every unaccounted pain or twinge in my body left me worried and concerned – a sort of cancer hypchondria. Gradually the fears lessened and while one never forgets, it ceased to dominate every day. I think it is a case of learning to live with the unpredictability of this particular disease and the realization that you could be on the bad side of the statistics chart. Of course, time does much to reassure you that you are, indeed, on the good side of that set of figures. And having faced that terror of cancer, you continue to live with even greater enjoyment, savoring the small things like dew on a spider web and the important large things like love for your husband and children, and in spite of sounding somewhat theatrical, these things have a greater meaning than before. I think it is important to point out that even then, in those darker days, and most certainly now, I have never had a moment of worry or doubt over the manner in which I was treated. Certainly, as I go about my daily activities, I have no constant physical reminder of the fact that I had cancer.

To be perfectly frank, I must tell you that the thought of speaking in public strikes terror in my heart, and I would not be here today if I did not feel it so important that more women understand that there are good medical choices on how cancer of the breast can be treated. Those of us in the medical field have a great opportunity because we are in the ideal position to help and assist countless women in making correct decisions regarding themselves. The most important thing of all in my estimation, is to spread the gospel of breast self-examination, particularly women, but men included since this particular cancer is not unknown among males. Examine yourself regularly and learn your own geography. Encourage others to do likewise. Most breast masses are discovered by the woman herself, an important fact to remember, because early detection raises the chances of cure. I stand here, a healthy and grateful five-year survivor because my lump was detected early and taken care of promptly and efficiently.

Fortunately, there is increased publicity in the media and some excellent articles have appeared recently in magazines, in newspapers and on television regarding the options, we, as patients, have regarding the treatment of cancer of the breast. Whereas four years ago, the phone calls I received were mainly from women, who for one reason or another, did not want to undergo even a modified radical mastectomy and were looking for advice on where to turn, now the largest percentage of calls are from women who have already made the decision to have a lumpectomy and radiation therapy and are seeking information on what to expect during the treatment. This is encouraging. Even some reach-to-recovery teams are able to give preoperative visits and discuss with the patient, alternate methods of treatment. And certainly, a symposium such as this does much to let the facts of the value of conservation surgery combined with radiation therapy be known. Perhaps if the knowledge could be shouted from the rooftops, my nineteen year old daughter would not have had to bring solace and comfort to her friend and classmate whose mother died from cancer of the breast, because, denying surgery, she knew of no alternative except holistic medicine.

Aurore Vaeth, RN, Mill Valley, CA 94941 (USA)

Front. Radiat. Ther. Onc., vol. 17, pp. 23–32 (Karger, Basel 1983)

Conservative Surgery and Radiation Therapy for Breast Cancer

Edmund L. Sacks, Offra G. Gerstein, Steven G. Mann

Stanford University Hospital and Medical Center, Palo Alto, Calif., USA

Medical Aspects

Introduction

The combination of breast-conserving surgery and radical radiation therapy is gaining acceptance as an alternative to mastectomy for primary breast cancer. Recent literature reports several hundred patients treated this way with local control and total survival comparable to more conventional treatment [1, 7, 19, 27, 36, 49, 52].

The major impetus for nonmastectomy therapy has emerged from large academic centers where many patients can be treated with consistent, albeit evolving techniques. The major beneficiaries of breast-saving therapies, however, are the patients who will ultimately be treated in their local communities, hopefully with techniques as sophisticated and results as good as those achieved in larger centers.

This report describes our experience in Santa Cruz County, California, from 1978 to 1981. During this time, we treated 37 women with breast cancer utilizing excisional surgery, external beam radiotherapy, and interstitial implant. We will present our techniques of treatment planning and therapy which can be performed in adequately equipped, community-based, radiotherapy facilities. In addition, we will report on a 1-year pilot project of psychological testing and concurrent group psychotherapy.

Materials and Methods

From May, 1978, to December, 1981, 37 women were treated with local excision followed by irradiation. These comprised 30% of all patients with regional localized breast cancer in northern Santa Cruz County. Ages ranged from 32 to 80 years. Patients were staged

Table I. Clinical staging

Stage I	
T_1N_0	21
Stage II	
T_1N_1	3
T_2N_0	7
T_2N_1	4
Stage III	
T_3	2
	—
	37

utilizing the system proposed by the American Joint Committee for Cancer Staging and End Results Reporting (table I). 2 patients with T_3 tumors were acceptable for treatment because total excision of the breast mass was feasible without serious deformation of the breast. In all cases, all grossly palpable disease was resected. 14 patients had axillary dissections; 8 had sampling of low axillary nodes only. The remaining 15 patients had no axillary investigation because they were postmenopausal and chemotherapy was not being considered as adjuvant treatment for them.

Treatment planning was originally performed by obtaining a contour utilizing a lead solder wire through the midplane of the breast. Since mid-1978, breast and chest wall thickness was determined utilizing the CT scanner. Since 1979, patients have undergone CT scanning in the treatment position to generate their contour as well as an isodose distribution from a Hewlett-Packard 9845B computer.

All patients except the initial 2 have been treated on a Varian Clinac 6/100, 6-MeV Linear Accelerator. The breast and chest wall were treated using medial and lateral opposed tangential or slightly angled fields at 100 cm SAD. Wedge filters were used for tissue compensation. The internal mammary chain, supraclavicular areas and axillary apex were treated in a single direct anterior field with the internal mammary chain portion eliminated in selected patients. Bolus was not used. Portal films were obtained to ensure that excess lung was not being treated. Treatment policy has been to treat all fields daily, with a modal dose of 180–200 rad to a total of 4,500 rad. Nodal areas at high risk have been treated with up to 5,000 rad.

33 patients have had interstitial implants to the excisional biopsy site using the ^{192}Ir afterloading technique. 3 patients refused the implant and one was medically unsuitable. It has been our practice in most cases to do at least a double-plane implant covering a generous portion of the resection site with a planned minimum tumor dose of 2,500 rad.

Of 21 patients who had axillary dissection or node sampling, 11 patients (53%) had positive nodes. 4 of these 11 (36%) were not appreciated on clinical examination. 1 woman with a clinically involved axillary node refused axillary surgery and subsequently received 6,500 rad to that node site. 10 out of 11 patients with positive nodes received concurrent adjuvant chemotherapy (table II).

Table II. Axillary status

	Dissection		Sampling	
	+	−	+	−
Clinically positive	6		1	
Clinically negative	1	6	3	4

Results

35 of 37 patients are alive and disease-free. 2 patients have relapsed and died. 1 of these patients had a highly anaplastic tumor; the other had a T_3 primary and, in retrospect, an equivocal bone scan prior to starting radiation therapy. With an average follow-up time of 16 months, there have been no local or regional recurrences.

Cosmetic results have been excellent with few exceptions. 3 patients undergoing axillary dissections have had prolonged, but mild, breast edema and increased breast tenderness following completion of therapy. 2 patients have developed mild telangiectasia and fibrosis at the site of the implant. Both had superficial single-plane implants in a flattened portion of the breast.

Discussion

Local excision followed by irradiation has now been reported by many institutions, including hundreds of patients, with follow-up of at least 4 years. Local control, regional control, and absolute survival are similiar when compared to patients treated by some form of mastectomy. Our series has an average follow-up of only 16 months, but so far, the local control rate (0/37 local failures) is consistent with other series.

Cosmetic results were excellent in most patients. Breast symmetry, absence of nipple disfigurement, and lack of skin color change except in the immediate implant area is characteristic. Often the treatment site could be identified in follow-ups only with careful examination. Factors which were important in giving good cosmetic results include: lack of bolus, boost with brachytherapy, external irradiation not greater than 5,000 rad, and surgery limited to excision of tumor (not quadrantectomy) in a plane not prone to cause breast retraction [6]. The brachytherapy boost should be given with sources placed no closer than 1 cm to the skin.

The equipment necessary to achieve good results should include supervoltage machine with X-rays generated at an energy of 1 MeV or greater. Energies of 10 MeV or greater should be avoided since the superficial tissues of the breast will be underdosed without bolus. Orthovoltage should never be used to treat the entire breast. [6].

In 1981, most patients in the USA treated for stage I and stage II breast cancer underwent modified radical mastectomies. The number of patient treated by lumpectomy and irradiation gradually has increased. 30 of the 37 patients in our series treated with lumpectomy and radiation were treated in the last 24 months. We expect the use of this technique to increase in our community during the next several years.

Psychologic Aspects

In recent years, there has been an increased awareness of the need to deal with the psychological factors in treatment of cancer patients [3, 5, 9, 15, 16, 23–25, 29, 31, 33, 34, 37–39, 41–43, 45–47, 51]. The need for a supportive milieu to help patients adjust has been emphasized in the care of stroke, cardiac and other medical groups [13, 28, 30, 48]. There have also been increasing amounts of data to suggest that with psychological support, patients heal faster and better [2, 4, 8, 10–12, 14, 18, 20–22, 26, 32, 35, 44, 50].

There were two main goals in developing this pilot project: (1) to provide a supportive environment to women who chose breast-saving procedure with radiation and (2) to develop research data based on these patients to determine their psychological profile and the benefits they may derive from the psychotherapeutic intervention. This project was funded by the Dominican Hospital Foundation of Santa Cruz.

Subjects, Methods and Materials

16 women between the ages of 35 and 58 participated in this program over the past year. All were within 1 week to a month past the diagnosis of breast cancer. All but 1 were married and all had children. These patients were referred by the radiation therapist. Out of 21 women who were offered this service 16 chose to partake in the counseling program. Out of the other 5, 3 felt too old and ill, 2 felt that they had sufficient support elsewhere. Since no further data are available regarding these 5 patients, it is not possible to compare them with those who chose to participate in group treatment. Two sequential groups of 8 women were conducted during the past year.

There were essentially four parts to this pilot project in which the patients participated and one relating to the contact between the psychologists and the radiation therapy staff. All patients underwent (1) an initial interview, (2) pretesting, (3) group psychotherapy and (4) posttesting.

Initial Interview. It covered the original family history, psychological, social and vocational adjustments and any current emotional difficulties.

Pretesting. Patients were administered four pretests: (a) MMPI, a standard measure of personality profile; Zung Depression Rating Scale, a short self-rating scale of 20 items dealing with both physical and psychological manifestations of depression; (c) Bem Sex Role Inventory, a self-scoring inventory based on internalized sex-typed behavior as masculine, feminine or androgynus; this was used to gain a measure of the women's level of assertiveness, aggression and self-reliance; (d) Bahnson's Anger Questionnaire, a 15-item questionnaire dealing with responses to anger from external striking out to internal self-punitive.

Group Psychotherapy. Patients joined a 2-hour weekly supportive group therapy. Each session consisted of two parts:
(a) Educational. A new topic was covered every week such as the psychological dynamics of stress, psychological effects of cancer diagnosis and treatment, dealing with anger, assertiveness within the context of healing, etc.
(b) Therapy. Sharing of feelings, support, openness of expression within the context of caring and intimacy.
Every 4 weeks the group therapy session included the patient's spouses. The husbands were given an opportunity to: share their feelings; deal with their fears, anger and disappointment about having temporarily lost a partner, and gained another child; a unique opportunity for these men to nurture and be nurtured by others who share the same experience.

Posttesting. After treatment, the women were administered the same tests as the pretesting with the omission of the MMPI and the addition of an open-ended questionnaire asking them to 'describe the changes they experienced which may be attributed to the group'.

Psychologist Radiation Therapy Staff Consultation. A periodic meeting between the psychologist and the radiotherapists and their staff allowed for better management of these patient's total adjustment to their cancer and treatment.

Results
The clinical interview revealed a group of women who seemed independent, competent, emotionally giving, with a uniqueness of mind yet, not very assertive. The choice of breast-saving procedure seemed to be the first major assertive act on their behalf.

The tests revealed that out of 16 MMPI profiles were normal. These women tended to deny unpleasantness in their lives and were likely to be seen by others as passive, agreeable and very 'good'. The other 4 women had less healthy personality profiles though their social and vocational adjustments were good.

On the Bem Sex Role Inventory, the women saw themselves prior to the diagnosis of cancer as basically happy, cheerful, positive about life, deferring to the needs of others, nonassertive and not depressed. After diagnosis and before group involvement, they reported being depressed and anxious a good part of the time, less cheerful, less hopeful, angry and fearful. After group therapy their profile resembled their prediagnosis of an improved disposition.

The Bahnson Anger Questionnaire and the Zen Depression Scale after group treatment revealed decreased levels of depression and anger, increased or regained sense of self-reliance and a stronger sense of hopefulness.

Group Therapy. In group treatment, it was interesting to note the various emotional struggles reported by these women. In addition to going through the trauma of the diagnosis of cancer and the associations attached to such diagnosis, these women also reported a few unique feelings for their particular condition and treatment.

(1) Insecurities regarding the decision to reject mastectomy and elect breast-saving procedure with radiation. Though the data and much medical research information support their choice, it nonetheless is taken at times quite trepidly. Women are not often used to making dramatic life-threatening decisions.

(2) Fear of recurrence which may jeopardize the wisdom of their choice of treatment was often discussed.

(3) Pressure from family and friends and other women who have chosen mastectomy is quite difficult to reconcile.

(4) Questions whether the treatment actually eradicated *all* cancer, since the breast is still there, are often raised with much need for reassurance and support from the other women.

(5) The implant: We were asked by a surgeon, 'Why do these women whose bodies are actually intact require so much support?' It is interesting to note that though these women suffer no permanent loss of body image, they experience similar body concerns regarding the implant.

– In spite of the fact that they receive detailed explanations with pictures and drawings from their radiation therapist and in spite of the fact that they hear about it from other patients, they still fear the radium implant procedure and have a strong sense of a temporary distortion of their body images during the time of the implant. The implant arouses extreme irrational fear about multilation. It seems to be the most traumatic part of treatment, both radiation and chemotherapy.

– Even though they suffer no permanent loss, there is also a fear of functional breast disfigurement due to the radiation procedure.

– Another frequent concern at the termination of treatment is the sense of abandonment. Lack of treatment is associated with lack of protection, renewed fears and a sense of vulnerability to recurrence of cancer.

Group therapy sessions allow these and other concerns to be aired and dealt with comfortably among women who share similar experiences and feelings.

Discussion

By both test results and women's reports, psychotherapy treatment in conjunction with medical treatment indicates several benefits. The women's abilities to reduce their anger, fear, hopelessness, and depression and increase their sense of assertiveness, hope, and well-being seem to accentuate the benefit of such combined treatment. The involvement of the patient's husband is a very important and valuable part of the treatment. Increased communication and intimacy ensued in all families. The exchange between the radiotherapy staff, physicians and the psychologists in a team approach helped patients be better cared for both medically and psychologically.

Conclusions

This pilot project was intended to provide both a service and a research data base for psychological profiles of women with primary breast cancer undergoing radiation. It met the first goal by indicating both by patients' reports and by test results that the support of a psychotherapy group assisted women in their adjustment to the disease and treatment and helped them in healing. It did not, however, provide control group comparisons. The second goal of obtaining psychological profiles was also accomplished. Yet, due to the small numbers involved, it does not allow for drawing board base conclusions. This, too, would require a tighter research design to determine whether these women differ from other women with breast cancer who have chosen mastectomy or no treatment.

This pilot project is now going into a second year with modified research design whereby some of the variables will be controlled and definite conclusions could be drawn as to the psychological nature of these patients, their treatment and possibility; even predictability of treatment benefits may be obtained.

The benefits of the service aspect of this psychological treatment in conjunction with radiotherapy has been shown to be valuable and is a viable program for patients in a small community-based practice.

References

1 Amahic, R.: Radiation therapy with or without primary limited surgery for operable breast cancer. Cancer *49:* 30–34 (1982).

2 Artiss, L.; Levine, S.: Doctor-patient relation in severe illness: a seminar for oncology fellows. New Engl. J. Med. *288:* 1210–1214 (1973).

3 Bahnson, C.: Psychologic and emotional issues in cancer: the psychotherapeutic care of the cancer patient. Semin. Oncol. *2:* 293–309 (1975).

4 Banister, O.K.; Dobos, J.A.: At-home rehab for cancer patients. Rehabil. *2:* 20–22 (1977).

5 Bard, M.; Sutherland, A.M.: Psychological impact of cancer and its treatment: IV. Adaptation to radical mastectomy. Cancer *8:* 656–672 (1955).

6 Bedwinek, J.: Treatment of stage I and II adenocarcinoma of the breast by tumor excision and irradiation. Int. J. Radiat. Oncol. Biol. Phys. *7:* 1553–1554 (1981).

7 Bourgeois, J.P.: Conservative treatment of cancers of the breast. Nouv. Presse Méd. *9:* 1242 (1980).

8 Cantor, R.: And a time to live: Toward emotional well-being during the crisis of cancer (Harper & Row, New York 1978).

9 Coppen, A.J.: Metcalf, M.: Cancer and extraversion; in Kissen, LeShan, Psychosomatic aspects of Neoplastic disease, pp. 30–34 (Lippincott, Philadelphia 1964).

10 Danaldson, M.H.: The multidisciplinary team approach to the care of children with cancer. Cancer Rev. *1/2:* 8–9 (1977).

11 Dorn, H.F.: Cancer and the marital status. Human. Biol. *15:* 73–79 (1943).

12 Feder, S.L.: Psychological considerations in the care of patients with cancer. Ann. N.Y. Acad. Sci. *125:* 1020–1027 (1966).

13 Friedman, S.B.; Glasgow, L.A.; Ader, R.: Psychosocial factors modifying host resistance to experimental infections. Ann. N.Y. Acad. Sci. *164:* 381–383 (1969).

14 Giacquinta, B.: Helping families face the crisis of cancer. Am. J. Nurs. *77:* 1585–1588 (1977).

15 Greene, W.A., Jr.: The psychosocial setting of the development of leukemia and lymphoma. Ann. N.Y. Acad. Sci. *125:* 794–801 (1966).

16 Greer, S.; Morris, T.: Psychological attributes to women who develop breast cancer. A controlled study. J. psychosom. Res. *19:* 147–153 (1975).

17 Guli, G., Jr.: The case for local excision of breast cancer in selected cases. Lancet: 549–551 (1972).

18 Halman, M.; Suttinger, J.: Family-center care for cancer patients. Nursing *78:* 42–43 (1978).

19 Harris, J.R., et al.: Primary radiation therapy for early breast cancer: the experience at the joint center for radiation therapy. Int. J.Radiat. Oncol. Biol. Phys. *7:* 1549–1552 (1981).

20 Healey, J.E., Jr.: Beyond definitive treatment: a new emphasis in cancer care. Postgrad. Med.: 214–218 (1970).

21 Henderson, I. W. D.: Psychological care of patients with malignant disease. Appl. Ther. *9:* 827–832 (1967).
22 Holland, J. C. B.: Psychological management of cancer patients and their families. Pract. Psychol.: 14–20 (1977).
23 Katz, J.; Gallagher, T.; Hellman, L.; Sachar, E.; Weiner, H.: Psychoendocrine considerations in cancer of the breast. Ann. N.Y. Acad. Sci. *164:* 509–516 (1969).
24 Klopfer, B.: Psychological variables in human cancer. J. project. Tech. *21:* 331–340 (1957).
25 LeShan, L. L.: A basic psychological orientation apparently associated with malignant disease. Psychiat. Q. *35:* 314 (1961).
26 Mantell, J. E.; Alexander, E. S.; Kleiman, M. A.: Social work and self-help groups. Health social Work *1:* 86–100 (1976).
27 Martinez, A.: Radical irradiation without a mastectomy.
28 Mastrovito, R. C.: Symposium: emotional considerations in cancer and stroke. N.Y. State J. Med. *72:* 2874–2877 (1972).
29 Meerlo, J.: Psychological implications of malignant growth: survey of hypotheses. Br. J. med. Psychol. *27:* 210–215 (1954).
30 Meerloo, J.: The initial neurologic and psychiatric picture syndrome of pulmonary growth. J. Am. med. Ass. *146:* 558–559 (1951).
31 Meyerowitz, B. E.; Sparks, F. C.; Spears, I. K.: Adjuvant chemotherapy for breast carcinoma: psychosocial implications. Cancer *43:* 1613–1618 (1979).
32 Miller, C. L.; Denner, P. R.; Richardson, V. E.: Assisting the psychosocial problems of cancer patients: a review of current research. Int. J. nurs. Students *13:* 161–166 (1976).
33 Muslin, H. L.; Gyarfas, K.; Pieper, W. J.: Separation experience and cancer of the breast. Ann. N.Y. Acad. Sci. *125:* 802–806 (1966).
34 Paloucek, F. P.; Graham, J. B.: The influence of psychosocial factors on the prognosis in cancer of the cervix. Ann. N.Y. Acad. Sci. *125:* 814–816 (1966).
35 Parsell, S.; Tagliareni, E. M.: Cancer patients help each other. Am. J. Nurs. *74:* 650–651 (1974).
36 Patterson, W. B.: Radiation therapy for primary breast cancer: some of the answers are in. Int. J. Radiat. Oncol. Biol. Phys. *7:* 1615–1616 (1981).
37 Psychophysiological Aspects of Cancer; in Weyer, Ann. N.Y. Acad. Sci. *125:* 773–1055 (1966).
38 Quint, J. C.: The impact of mastectomy. Am. J. Nurs. *63:* 83–92.
39 Reznikoff, J.: Psychological factors in breast cancer: a preliminary study of some personality trends in patients with cancer of the breast. Psychosom. Med. *18:* 2 (1955).
40 Richter, M., et al.: The role of axillary sampling in the primary radiation therapy of primary breast cancer (Ab 59). Proc. Am. Ass. Cancer Res. *21:* 414 (1980).
41 Schmale, A. H.; Iker, H.: Hopelessness as a predictor of cervical cancer. Soc. Sci. Med. *5:* 95–100 (1971).
42 Schmale, A. H.: Psychological reactions to recurrence, metastases, or disseminated cancer. Radiat. Oncol. Biol. Phys. *1:* 515–520 (1976).
43 Senescu, R. A.: The development of emotional complications in the patient with cancer. J. chron. Dis. *16:* 813–832 (1963).
44 Sheldon, A.; Shih, D.; Ryser, C. P.; Krant, M. J.: An integrated family oriented cancer care program: the report of a pilot project in the socio emotional management of chronic disease. J. chron. Dis. *22:* 743–755 (1977).

45 Solomon, G. F.: Emotions, stress, the central nervous system and immunity. Ann. N.Y. Acad. Sci. *164:* 333–343 (1966).
46 Southam, C. M.: Discussion: emotions immunology, and cancer: how might the psyche influence neoplasia? Ann. N.Y. Acad. Sci. *164:* 473–475 (1966).
47 Stavraky, K. M.: Psychological factors in the outcome of human cancer. J. psychosom. Res. *12:* 251 (1968).
48 Thomas, C. B.; Duszynski, D. R.: Closeness to parents and the family constellation in a prospective study of five disease states: suicide, mental illness, malignant tumor, hypertension, and coronary heart disease. Johns Hopkins med. J. *134:* 251–270 (1974).
49 Vilcoq, J. R., et al.: The outcome of treatment by tumorectomy and radiotherapy of patients with operable breast cancer. Int. J. Radiat. Oncol. Biol. Phys. *7:* 1327–1332 (1981).
50 Waxenberg, S. E.: The importance of the communications of feelings about cancer. Ann. N.Y. Acad. Sci. *125:* 1000–1055 (1966).
51 Wheeler, J. I., Jr.; Caldwell, B. R.: Psychological evaluation of women with cancer of the breast and of the cervix. Psychosom. Med. *17:* 256–268 (1955).
52 Wise, L., et al.: Local excision and irradiation: an alternative method for the treatment of early mammary cancer. Ann. Surg. *174:* 392–400 (1971).

E. L. Sacks, MD, Santa Cruz, Radiation Oncology Medical Group, Stanford University Hospital and Medical Center, Palo Alto, CA (USA)

Front. Radiat. Ther. Onc., vol. 17, pp. 33–40 (Karger, Basel 1983)

The Patient's Right to Know under the Law

Matthew B. Weinberg

West Coast Cancer Foundation, San Francisco, Calif., USA

Our nation functions under the rule of law, not under the rule of man. Our rights, duties, and consequent responsibilities are derived from the law.

This is what makes our system acceptable to the people of our great nation and why we have endured under the same system for more than 200 years.

The law is derived generally from the legislative process, the administrative rule-making process, and the application of *stare decisis*. Against this background, we examine a particular law passed in California in an attempt to assure that a patient will know the alternatives for treating breast cancer. By way of legislative history, this California law derives initially from the legislative process; but to become effective, it will have to be filtered through the administrative bureaucracy, which I referred to as the rule-making process.

The California statute which is intended to satisfy the patient's right to know about alternatives for treating breast cancer is largely the result of one woman's reaction to what she found to be a particularly insensitive physician. The patient in question lay in her hospital bed after undergoing tests because she had noticed blood exuding from the nipple of her right breast. By telephone, her physician gave her the news that she had breast cancer and according to her account, without explanation told her that he had reserved an operating room for early the next morning because she would have to have a major operation. When the physician explained to her what her operation, a modified radical mastectomy, was, the patient was appalled. She feared disfigurement, weakening of her arm muscles, and that the possibility of restorative plastic surgery would be difficult, if not impossible. And most of all, as she testified in legislative hearings months later, she was angry because the surgeon had offered no explanation of why he felt the operation was essential, or what other options might be available.

Under these circumstances, the patient cancelled her surgeon's orders, rejected the operation, and saw one cancer specialist after another to seek alternatives that might give her an equal chance of survival and be less drastic, both physically and psychologically. Among the alternatives that were ultimately explained to her was removing little more than the lump in the breast, plus her under arm lymph nodes, to be followed by radiation therapy to destroy any invisible cancer tissue in the breast. This latter course, the lumpectomy, was chosen by the patient, who, after the surgery healed and her radiation therapy had been completed, found that her breast began to return to its normal size and shape. When it was over, the patient was angry. She realized that only by her own force of will had she been spared the more radical procedure.

It was then that she decided there ought to be a law about this. She turned to her State Senator, David Roberti, and insisted that he introduce a bill which would compel physicians and surgeons to inform breast cancer patients about all treatment options in advance, so the patient can participate fully in the decision-making process as to the method of treatment, not merely as to the decision of whether or not to accept a proposed treatment.

Of course, one person does not a law make, so the patient started a movement that gathered strength from the growing number of consumer activists in the health care field, and the pressure was on. Senator Roberti and a group of Senate colleagues finally pushed a bill through the Legislature in September of 1980, over the opposition, amongst others, of the California Medical Association and most lobbying medical groups.

What is this law that the California Legislature passed? It was Health and Safety Code Section 1704.5, adopted in the 1980 Legislative Session and effective on January 1, 1981. It provides that the failure of a physician or surgeon to inform a patient by means of a standardized written summary, which is to be developed by the Department of Health Services and the Cancer Advisory Council, of the alternative efficacious methods of treatment of breast cancer constitutes unprofessional conduct. The statute requires that the standardized written summary be in layman's language understood by the patient, and that the standardized written summary be printed and made available by the Board of Medical Quality Assurance to physicians and surgeons. This written summary must set forth the advantages, disadvantages, risks, and descriptions of the procedures with regard to medically viable and efficacious alternative methods of treatment.

Actually, under the law, all the physician has to do is give this written summary to the patient. To do so constitutes compliance with the law; failure to do so constitutes unprofessional conduct.

What do we mean by unprofessional conduct? Under Sections 2257, 2221, and 2227 of the California Business and Professions Code, unprofessional conduct may be grounds for a physician to have his certificate to practice medicine revoked, suspended, or denied, or may result in probation or public reprimand. However, these actions can only take place after the physician is found guilty in a disciplinary proceeding. Some other examples of unprofessional conduct under the Code, include being intoxicated while treating patients, furnishing drugs to a patient without a good faith prior examination, and failing to comply with rules of informed consent for sterilization procedures.

The key point to emphasize regarding this statute is that the Legislature, in effect, has only acted to compel the physician to distribute the standardized written summary to the patient. But the Legislature deems that important enough so that the penalty for failure to do so could be loss of the right to practice medicine.

Interestingly, the statute does not require the physician to explain the alternative methods of treatment and does not require any explanation of the balance of risks and benefits. Likewise, it does not contemplate any civil penalties for non-compliance. As such, it in no way replaces the independent duty of the physician to obtain a patient's informed consent prior to undertaking medical or surgical treatment.

This is as far as the Legislature has taken this matter.

As of the date of this Symposium there are no regulations adopted in connection with this statute, and though it has gone through approximately 23 drafts, the standardized written summary required to be produced by the Board of Medical Quality Assurance still has not been printed after more than 15 months since the passage of the statute. The law therefore is stalled at the stage of the administrative process.

It is interesting to study what other states have done in this area. By way of comparison, a bill was signed into law in May of 1979, as Chapter 214 of the Commonwealth of Massachusetts Statutes entitled 'The Commonwealth's Patient's Rights Act.' It took effect on August 21, 1979. This act pertains only to patients who are treated in a health care facility. This statute is intended as a patient's bill of rights. It establishes that the patient has actionable rights once admitted to a health care facility. For example, the patient has the right to informed consent (in California, the doctrine arises under the common law), the patient has the right to privacy during medical treatment, the right to refuse to be examined, the right to refuse to serve in a research project. In addition, there is tagged onto this patient bill of rights a section which says:

> 'In the case of a patient suffering from any form of breast cancer, [the patient has the right] to complete information on all alternative treatments which are medically viable, and any person whose rights under this section are violated may bring, in addition to any other action allowed by law, a civil action under sections [of the Massachusetts Act].'

The statutes of Massachusetts and California each speak in terms of the patient being informed of medically viable treatment alternatives. But the statutes differ in that the Massachusetts statute establishes this as a patient right and provides civil penalties for failure to comply with this right. The California statute on the other hand establishes a physician's duty to deliver a written document to his patient. Failure to carry out this duty can result in professional disciplinary measures, but there is no new civil right of action given to the patient. I leave you to ponder on that dichotomy.

Other experts at this Symposium will deal with the medical questions underlying the reason why some members of the profession do not accept the lumpectomy as a viable medical alternative to more radical surgical procedures. But since this appears to be the case today, the California Legislature, through its popularist process, shall require every physician and surgeon, no matter what his individual opinion may be, to present a written summary arrived at by committee to each patient.

There may be great wisdom in the requirement of a written summary. Since to explain an alternative method of treatment which a physician or surgeon does not believe to be proven may be as discouraging and confusing to the patient as not to reveal it at all. Under the California system, when the patient sees the written summary, the patient will at least have the alternative or opportunity to turn to another specialist for advice on the form of treatment.

Another interesting comparison to consider is between the California statute and the doctrine of informed consent in California. Informed consent rather than having its roots in the legislative process is the result of the judicial process and the judiciary's application of the common law tort of battery. Battery is the unauthorized touching of another without his permission. The Courts found that most medical procedures constitute an actionable battery in the absence of consent. Informed consent is the patient's permission to perform a procedure or test after he has a sufficient understanding of what he is consenting to. Informed consent is summarized in a landmark 1972 California Supreme Court decision entitled *Cobbs v. Grant*. In this case, the Supreme Court stated: 'In sum, the patient's right of self-decision is the measure of the physician's duty to reveal. That right can be effectively exercised only if the patient possesses adequate information to enable an intelligent choice. The scope of the physician's communications to the patient then must be measured by the patient's need, and that need is whatever information is material to the decision. Thus, the test for determining whether a potential peril must be divulged is its materiality to the patient's decision.'

As you can see, we attorneys do not write any more clearly than most physicians write on their prescription pads. In more straight-forward terms, what the Court was saying in *Cobbs* was the following: Patients are generally medically unknowing, and doctors are supposedly medically knowledgeable. Patients have the right to control their own body and determine whether or not to submit to a treatment. For a patient to do so, he must give consent based upon information provided to him by the doctor. Because this abject dependence is combined with general trust in the doctor, there arises a fiduciary duty of the physician to the patient. The fiduciary duty must be discharged with reasonable disclosure of available choices with respect to the proposed treatment, of the dangers inherent and potentially involved in the treatment, and of the probability of successful outcome of the treatment. The scope of duty to disclose may be measured, amongst other things, by the amount of knowledge the patient needs in order to make an informed choice. This standard, of course, is subjective, depending upon who the patient is, his level of knowledge, and what his concerns are. But in any event, all information material to treatment and the patient's condition should be disclosed. 'Material' means facts not commonly appreciated and which would be regarded as significant by a reasonable person. Failure to discharge this fiduciary duty to the patient is the basis for civil liability of the professional to the patient. It can be argued that the explanation of alternative forms of treatment is information material to treatment and must be disclosed under the doctrine of informed consent.

The California breast cancer legislation differs quite markedly from the approach of informed consent. At most, the cancer legislation adopted in California would put the patient on notice to seek more advice. Breast cancer legislation as adopted in Massachusetts goes hand in hand with the patient's right to the information required under the law for informed consent, and as pointed out earlier, the requirements of informed consent are part of the patient's rights under the Massachusetts statute. The California legislation in no way replaces the common law duty of a physician to obtain the patient's informed consent prior to undertaking a medical or surgical treatment. To be sure, failure to comply with the California statute provides strong evidence of a lack of informed consent for purposes of civil suit, while following the statute to the letter without doing more will not absolve the physician of the obligation to obtain the patient's informed consent after explaining the alternatives available. In this respect, the statute provides a sword for the patient, but no shield for the physician.

Now, I turn to a very brief analysis of some benefits and problems arising from this law.

Cancer is a life-threatening condition, and presents to most victims their most important health care decision. It is frightening, and it is difficult. Therefore, it is easy to understand the problems that the California legislation presents to draftsmen of the written summary. The draftsmen must take into consideration and account the fact that the patient finds herself in this life-threatening condition, having to make an important decision. The draftsmen must present choices which, in some cases, may not even be readily available, and to some persons, may, by themselves, be a source of great fright. Therefore, one of the great problems of this legislation is its implementation.

The most obvious benefit of this legislation is with respect to the surgeon who did not present viable treatment alternatives to the patient, such as the doctor described in the history of the legislation. There is the question of whether that kind of problem was so widespread as to justify developing the written summary. Nevertheless, I think most will agree that as to those physicians and surgeons who did not present the various alternatives to their recommended treatment, that the written summary will solve a problem. I would like to discuss several other positive and negative aspects of this approach to the patient's rights.

The requirement of reducing to a reviewable written form, a layman's description of these matters is intriguing. There are reams of material on the professional level, utilizing professional jargon, to describe diagnosis and treatment of breast cancer. Under the doctrine of informed consent, the health care professional is required to translate and communicate this material to the patient. Each patient has been subject to her individual doctor's extent of knowledge, to her individual doctor's ability as a communicator, and to her individual doctor's personal judgments and opinions (which proponents of this legislation described as their prejudices). The written summary may result in patient material which overcomes the weaknesses in an individual physician's knowledge, ability to communicate, or prejudices. Juxtaposed against this advantage is the problem of presenting alternatives which may be medically viable in some situations, but not in others, which may create confusion when the patient considers the standardized summary and the ultimate recommendations of her treating physician.

Another serious problem is how to keep a standardized written summary up to date, once it is completed. What does the physician or surgeon do with his breast cancer patient during the interim period from the time that the summary becomes outdated and a substitute summary is developed. If it takes 15 plus months to prepare the initial summary, it may take 15 plus months to obtain a concensus on changing the summary.

Under the law, the physician would still be required to deliver the summary to avoid being guilty of unprofessional conduct. Will the use of an out-of-date summary be misleading; will the physician have to tell the patient that certain portions of the brochure no longer state the best medical view on the treatments described? Will such statements by the physician violate the law? Is the Board of Medical Quality Assurance authorized to withdraw a statement?

These are questions which arise from the California approach to the problem.

Another question this leads to is will we have to create a bureaucracy which will be required to write summaries to translate complex medical knowledge into summary written form understandable to laymen? I raise this last point because if the standardized written summary is the most effective method of informing patients of what they have the right to know, why limit it to breast cancer patients?

Today, there is much discussion of whether there are too many bypass surgeries, and most recently, as to whether there are too many cesarean surgeries. True, a radical mastectomy disfigures the patient's sexual image, but is this more severe or more dangerous than open-heart surgery? Therefore, a major question we face is: Is there any medical reason to require a standardized summary for the treatment of breast cancer and not require a similar summary in other dread diseases and conditions?

From a jurisprudential point of view, to limit the approach to breast cancer is to have enacted special-interest legislation which gives one group more solicitous treatment under by the law than the population as a whole receives when it faces other difficult medical choices.

Part of the answer to these questions may come in an analysis of the extent to which a patient should place his or her reliance and trust upon a professional and his professional opinion, and the extent to which it is desirable for the patient afflicted with a life-threatening disease or condition to himself or herself become an expert on that disease or condition.

In conclusion, the written summary, once available, will benefit those patients who are under the care of the few insensitive and arrogant physicians and surgeons who have not informed their patients about alternative methods of treatment. But is this a great enough benefit? I hope I leave you with more questions than answers, because, at this point, the California legislation appears to raise more interesting questions than the number of problems it solves.

M. B. Weinberg, MD, West Coast Cancer Foundation, San Francisco, CA 94104 (USA)

Front. Radiat. Ther. Onc., vol. 17, pp. 41–47 (Karger, Basel 1983)

Discussion

Alan Schroeder (Moderator): We heard from Dr. *Kelly* about the emotional traumas which not only the patient might have but the family of the patient might have. I wonder if there isn't a group of patients who perhaps are not suitable, perhaps from a psychiatric point of view as well as from a risk factor. I allude to those patients who develop a lesion, and as she said in her opening remarks, may have had relatives who when they were premenopausal had bilateral breast cancer. Perhaps they should be considered for a procedure other than tylectomy and radiation therapy.

The presentation from Santa Cruz was most intriguing. Dr. *Sacks* mentioned that he has irradiated patients with axillary nodes who were undergoing concurrent chemotherapy. What were the reactions? Were they able to handle these reactions? The psychotherapy study that they are doings is quite unique, and I would like to hear more about it. I wonder if the patients that they are seeing in Santa Cruz are perhaps in a different group than we see in other areas. Santa Cruz may have a socioeconomic status which allows patients to seek out this kind of therapy. Has this been looked at? It seems that the group of patients who selected to be seen in psychotherapy had a great deal of homogeneity characteristics

Dr. Sacks (Santa Cruz, Calif.): Those patients who had chemotherapy generally had a cycle of chemotherapy prior to initiating the radiation therapy. If their blood counts tolerated it, and most did, they received full dose chemotherapy during the course of the irradiation. We really didn't notice any additional skin reaction that I could attribute to the combination chemotherapy/radiation therapy. We're using 6-MeV photons which may be responsible for this. There has been slightly more erythema in the supraclavicular area, but all our patients seem to have that reaction, with or without chemotherapy. We've seen no additional acute reactions. We're seeing more telangiectasis of the breast around the implant on the chemotherapy patients. Perhaps this is due to my technique, or due to the combination therapy.

Our patient population is pretty much evenly divided between premenopausal and postmenopausal women. Santa Cruz is a retirement community, at least it has been in the past. Most of the patients that we have treated are actively doing something – they're teaching, working in some respect, or active housewives. I'm not sure that there has been any selection from that standpoint. There has definitely been a selection in which surgical groups refer to our practice. One group of surgeons doesn't like doing mastectomies and considers them mutilating procedures.

Schroeder: What chemotherapeutic agents were you using during radiation therapy, and were they getting full doses?

Sacks: CMF, and they were getting full doses, and their blood counts tolerated it.

Schroeder: And how long was that continued?

Sacks: Generally for a year. My experience in Santa Cruz is only 3 years.

Jack Sherman (San Francisco, Calif.): In counseling patients for either surgery or definitive radiation for their breast cancer, physicians commonly list the more routine complications. What do you think is appropriate in terms of informed consent with respect to the less common complications?

Mr. Weinberg (San Francisco, Calif.): Informed consent, which is complex, puts the duty on you as physician to discuss with your patient and describe to your patient the benefits, problems, conditions, results as measured by the standards of the area in which you practice.

Sherman: Let me expand on that. What I was getting at was that if you have a woman who refuses mastectomy, and you're going to offer her radiation therapy, if you counsel her thoroughly enough to everything that could possibly happen, she won't accept radiation therapy either. How much is one required to emphasize? For example, the rarest problem, the one that we worry about that we usually don't tell the patient, is the extremely unlikely possibility of inducing a second malignancy from the irradiation. Now many people would feel if you tell the patient who is already terrified that it could happen, then they will not choose radiation therapy; and yet they have already rejected mastectomy. Where do you draw the line legally? You can say, 'Well, the community standard', but the standard in San Francisco is very variable in terms of what patients are told.

Weinberg: I would make two points. The first is that you are expressing a very subjective conclusion which may be based upon your experience that these are the things that if I tell them they won't do what I think they should do, and these are the things which I think I can afford to tell them without discouraging them from doing that. What you are, in effect, saying goes against the doctrine of informed consent which is that you ultimately should be making the decision for the patient as the treatment to be accepted. The doctrine of informed consent really requires that the patient have laid out before her all of the aspects of the treatments and the reasons for it and the results of it, and then that patient is to make a decision, albeit a decision contrary to the one the physician might have made, but the patient's own decision. Whether that's good or bad notwithstanding, that is the doctrine of informed consent. The second point I would make deals with a very interesting and recent case which I didn't go into in my presentation but really relates to what you're saying. It's a unique case recently in California in which the physician had recommended a Pap test to his patient. The patient had not taken the Pap test. The patient developed cancer of the cervix, the patient expired, and suit was brought. The defense was the physician had recommended a Pap test to the patient. The case was lost by the physician on the basis that the physician had failed to fully explain the effect of not taking the Pap test and what could occur in those instances. So once again you're put to the standard of explaining to the patient as best you can all of the aspects of the matter that you are dealing with, as well as the things that can go wrong if the patient doesn't undertake the treatment. This is a very different kind of case because it doesn't deal with battery at all, as you can see. It was recommended to the patient to take the test, the patient didn't take the test, there was no treatment, there was no touching. Nevertheless, the court, in effect, found that it was negligent not to have explained in detail all of the aspects that are important for the patient to know.

Cantril (San Francisco, Calif.): I would like to address a question to Mrs. *Vaeth* and then one to Mr. *Weinberg.* I personally abhor the idea of legislating medical care. I find that it's inconsistent with the practice and profession of medicine, and I also think that it is going to come up with all sorts of problems that can't be resolved, such as the one Mr. *Weinberg* said when the technology changes and we have to wait 2 or 3 years to get a new regulation. However, the question to Mrs. *Vaeth* is really: What do your feel – I know you're already very informed and were prior to the time of even considering breast cancer – nonetheless, do you think that a standardized piece of paper handed out by your surgeon would have been helpful?

Mrs. Vaeth (Mill Valley, Calif.): Perhaps not in my own particular case. It would seem to me that a bona fide piece of paper with all the details of treatment options probably would not carry the bias that a physician who was informing the person might convey. I don't think it is the whole answer either. I think it's a start.

Cantril: Mr. *Weinberg,* if a female client of yours comes to you and says, 'Mr. Weinberg, I think I have breast cancer, and I'm going to talk to my physicians about it', would you advise her that you go with her to talk to her physicians?

Weinberg: No, I wouldn't advise her that I go with her in the sense that her physician has the same fiduciary responsibility and duty to the patient as her attorney does. Therefore, in her communications and dealings with her attorney, she should be able to deal with complete faith and confidentiality with her attorney. I would't think it would be necessary for me to go with her to such a proceeding. However, if the patient comes away confused, upset or distressed, now I think she can afford to go see her attorney, because legislature has gotten involved, as you said, in the practice of medicine. Once the legislature gets involved, the attorneys get involved. That's why legislators, most of whom are attorneys, are so good at making so many laws. Now if your attorney who has long had a place in this field with respect to the question of negligence, malpractice, and the like, will have an even further place, I don't know. Now we have a question of whether the license should be lifted for failure to comply with the law. I think the attorney is going to have a greater place, but I don't think he needs to become involved in the patient's direct dealings with her physicians until a complaint has arisen.

Lawton (Hampton, Iowa): Dr. *Sacks,* I am aware that adjuvant therapy is popular. I am also aware that there is an increased disease-free interval, but I am also further aware that the survival of patients has not been proved to be increased by the use of chemotherapy as an adjuvant to radiotherapy. I was wondering why you use it, especially when you've controlled the local disease, and we're not sure you can control distant spread with adjuvant therapy.

Sacks: The complete discussion of adjuvant chemotherapy is beyond the scope of my presentation. However, this is not a direct answer to your question, which would take an entire symposium to answer. We generally practice to the standards that are practiced elsewhere in Northern California, and the standard practice in most of the rest of Northern California was to treat pre- and perimenopausal women with positive axillary nodes with chemotherapy. I leave that decision up to the medical oncologist, and we make that decision as a team. We tend to approach a lot of diseases in Santa Cruz that way, and our best available knowledge in the past several years has been that chemotherapy does improve the disease-free interval in patients where it is generally indicated. I don't think there is any magic in CMF chemotherapy. That's my own personal belief. But the standard of treatment during this time period was to do that, and that was considered the best available therapy. That's what our ladies received.

Richard Lowy (Portland, Oreg.): I have been very interested in the economic considerations and have had very little dialogue or information as to how the surgeon and the radiotherapist interact in this area. Obviously a mastectomy is a far more lucrative procedure than a tylectomy and lymph node dissection, and I wonder if any of you have ever discussed this as surgeons or heard discussions about this, and how this may influence your judgement. Somehow I think it is influencing the practice of medicine as much as the surgeon's and radiotherapist's own ego structures.

Sacks: I don't have the actual RVS numbers, but I think the total fee for a formal axillary dissection as well as a lumpectomy is almost as much as the modified radical mastectomy.

Lowy: Have you ever asked the surgeon his fees?

Sacks: I've never pointedly asked the question, 'What are the actual charges?' In terms of what the actual costs are for the two different treatments, if you exclude patients getting postoperative radiation after a mastectomy, but just comparing mastectomy versus breast conservation, I actually think our procedure is more expensive, particularly when you put in the cost of the iridium, which is several hundreds of dollars, and the implant procedure. That's one reason we started doing it on an outpatient basis under local anesthesia, and also in several cases have done it at the time the lymph node dissection was performed. We try to cut costs in that way, but I think ultimately our method costs more than a mastectomy.

Weinberg: I think that raises some interesting questions which are related to the direct question which I would perhaps deal with by saying that most doctors I've met have always said the one thing they didn't teach them in medical school was how to charge, how to bill and what the fees should be. Maybe that's an indication of what they should be considering when they make a medical decision, that those really are not factors, except to this extent, and that's where I wanted to comment. The problem with ever presenting all viable alternatives is, can they always be applied in each instance? I'll give a couple of examples. One is the question of the patient who lives 250 miles from the nearest radiation therapy treatment center. What does she do if she wants to choose an alternative of lumpectomy and radiation therapy, and she lives on a farm with 7 children? Does she drive 250 miles each way every day? Does she stay in a motel in the area of the radiation therapy treatments center, leaving her family alone for a period of 4–8 weeks, whatever the treatment series is going to be? Or does she go ahead and have her breast removed in the local hospital? These kinds of questions I think are real, and I think the professional should be aware of them and be sensitive to them. The other aspect of it is what are the various costs of treatment, what kind of coverage does the patient have, and, therefore, what can the patient afford to do? I think you raised some interesting questions.

John Cherry (La Jolla, Calif.): As a surgeon, I would like to answer the economic question. When modified radical mastectomy emerged, it proved to be more work at the operating table to effect a good axillary dissection, and it proved to be as much or more trouble postoperatively caring for the patient's long range. The RVS schedule listed modified radical mastectomies at a lesser fee than radical mastectomy. Nevertheless, the majority of surgeons have turned to modified radical mastectomy. The RVS schedules for a modified axillary dissection and wide local excision of the breast mass approaches that of a modified radical mastectomy. I think it's inappropriate and abhorrent that any physicians would base their treatment upon the RVS schedule and its magnitude.

Campbell (La Jolla, Calif.): We did a cost analysis of our first 30 cases, thanks mostly to *John Cherry,* who refers most of our patients, and the total cost for the radiation therapy procedure, including anesthesia, our own admission to the hospital (we admit all of our own patients) was under $5,000. That's a year ago, perhaps, and I suspect that's escalated to around $5,700. I'm a Scotsman, and I assure you that includes everything that the patient spent because I think it's a procedure that should not be cost-controlled or concerned. I think if we're going to compete with the surgeons, which we are doing, it's nice to be able to tell a patient from day one if they ask or even if they don't ask what's the cost involved, and we can tell them what it costs at our institution. It's under $ 6,000 today completely, including the radioactive seeds and the physics.

Mike Levine (Orinda, Calif.): One has to consider in the total cost of the mastectomy procedure the potential costs of reconstructive surgery which most women in our locale would opt to have if they underwent mastectomy. It is my own personal opinion when you add the psychological costs to the total cost of surgery that the radiation technique with tylectomy is a very cost-effective procedure compared to any other approach.

Helen Caruthers (San Francisco, Calif.): I'm with the California Division of the American Cancer Society, and I found the attorney's presentation most interesting, although I think I'm more confused now than before I came. For those of us who have been involved in providing input to the state on the development of the standard information, I think we see the difficulty of their task, and most of us would rather see a different approach toward the problem. The people in this room are probably those who provide far better communication than a lot of the physicians who should be here and are not. I think those are the physicians to which the law is really addressed. I wanted to mention that the California Division granted a study on the psychosocial needs of cancer patients in California in 1979, and among some of the interesting findings one of the most pointed was that at the time of diagnosis, one of the most critical needs of patients was communication, or should I say the lack of communication, between patient and physician, not really knowing what was going on. We really have to keep in perspective the void at that point and that the law may not be the best way to meet that, but it has not been met in several ways. We have seen books written – in fact, there is an author in this room, *Mary Spletter,* who has just written a book called *A Woman's Choice* published by Beacon Press, that I think is one more step in the direction of patients really taking into their own hands the need to inform their peers about information and options at this point in time. We have to keep that in perspective. Generally in our 'Reach to Recovery Program', we see time and again at the point following diagnosis that patients have not really been provided the kind of basic information that they need, and were there some other way to go about it, it would be nice, but at this point the law is upon us, and we have to cope with it.

Prosnitz (New Haven, Conn.): Mr. *Weinberg,* I have a brief question. Who is writing the California information sheet?

Weinberg: Well, here are some specific names. The document is being prepared by the California Health Services Department. Dr. *Sherwood Lawrence,* who I think is participating here in this symposium today, is one of the principal persons responsible for the ultimate drafting of the document. I've gone over several of the most recent drafts, and I find it a very interesting and difficult project. Nevertheless, as I pointed out in my presentation, this is intriguing. Perhaps it's a good idea; let's see how we can come out with putting this down on paper in layman's terms. The greatest advantage I see at this point is the fact that in forcing it to be put down on paper it becomes reviewable. Once it becomes reviewable, we can begin to discuss it. Whereas what the doctor is saying in his own office with the patient regarding informed consent is not reviewable.

Prosnitz: We wrote such a document and have been giving it to our patients at Yale for about a half a dozen years or so, but it needs frequent revisions, as you pointed out. I think your last comment in your formal talk was perhaps the most revealing and the one which I would agree with you – you phrased it politely and said that the California legislation perhaps raises more questions and problems than it solves. I think I would change the wording just a little bit and say that it seems to raise more problems than it's going to solve. I say that as one who has been an advocate – I don't like to use the word 'advocate' – but let's say one who has talked about and had some interest in this area for a number of years. Still, I don't think we are going to solve the problem of informing patients through the state legislature. There is another word in the presentation, and that was that the patient had to be informed about the known efficacy or efficaciousness of treatment. Again this kind of thing changes quite frequently.

Sherwood Lawrence (Calif.): I'm a physician, and I was in private individual practice for quite a while before I became a bureaucrat. I'd like to congratulate Mr. *Weinberg* on his presentation. It was very empathetic, and I think it's very appropriate the remarks has made about the difficulty of preparing such a draft. We are not required to quantitate the efficaciousness of any of these procedures. We simply have to classify whether or not a procedure is viable and efficacious, and we are supposed to write a written summary of them. Our problems are just to do that – to show their advantages and disadvantages. It has been very difficult; as you can recognize there is not even total agreement amongst physicians who are radiotherapists, there is not total agreement amongst surgeons who are just amongst themselves. When you get the two groups together and then add medical oncologists, a consensus of the medical profession in this field is a very basic, very difficult thing to achieve. We worked out a compromise, you might say, with the aid of very thoughtful input from many parts of the profession. We felt we had complied with the requirements of the act which the legislature put through and the governor signed, but we have a compunction of a feeling that we have toward the senator who originated the legislation to agree that it meets the requirements of his bill. We have found through a series of misadventures that the senator and his advocates had a particular thought in mind when they introduced the legislation, but by the time the medical profession through the CMA had expressed themselves sufficiently in the passage through the legislature, that the bill came out with not what they had in mind. We are in the position of having to write a document that responds to the law, but we are trying to get it written in such a fashion that Senator Roberti and his advocates are satisfied, it meets their requirements which are not in the law. So we have been delayed somewhat. We would like to emphasize, as Mr. *Weinberg* has said, that this is not to replace informed consent. We have tried to make the presentation in the brochure that we are writing up sufficiently balanced so that when a surgeon presents it to the patient he is going to say, 'These are the facts as required by the law, and I have to give it to you', and not have him say, 'Here's this piece of paper the damn state requires us to give you. It's full of prejudice and nonsense, but I am required by law to give it to you or lose my license.' We'd also have the same problem with radiotherapists if we made it prejudiced in favor or surgery. I think it's extemely important to point out what you are all aware of, and that is that the entry into the radiation therapists is through the chamber of the surgeons. And this is a process of evaluation going on which is causing problems where there are surgeons like the lady down in Beverly Hills had. I think the legislation will ameliorate that problem. I think it will make the approach which Dr. *Sacks* is experiencing in Santa Cruz increase. I hope that in the long run we will be able to get a device out which will get past the senators – we are meeting with them Monday again – and get it in the field. There is no provision in the law to update it. We have tried to construct it and phrase it so that it is stated as kind of a basic situation. We have tried to make it open – ended enough so that the patient in discussing the matter with her surgeon, family physician, radiotherapist, medical oncologist, gynecologist, or whomever, will got to that person of other persons that her physician may recommend for additional information. We have tried to orient the whole thing to the fact that the patient is going to learn the ABC's, but to find out what really goes on, she has to go to a special source. We have delineated her right to chose a different physician or to request consultation, and the right of her physician to withdraw from the case if he is not satisfied with her decision or to refer her or to seek additional consultation for their mutual benefit. There are probably some other features I haven't mentioned, but it's been a tough job, and I do hope it's about over.

Dr. Levitt (Minneapolis, Minn.): I'd like to ask Mr. *Weinberg* if he or anybody else in the audience has any information as to how effective the law in Massachusetts has been. The reason I am asking is that right now in the Minnesota legislature there is a proposal for instituting a similar piece of legislation, and I think one of the measures is the efficacy. I don't know how you measure efficacy in something like this.

Weinberg: I don't have an answer, but I will say this about the Massachusetts law. It will, to some extent, be self-policing because it gives the patients rights, and the patient can then exercise those rights. It's a long drawn-out process to the extent that to exercise those rights through the judicial process takes a period of years. I did not seek to determine whether there have been any judicial determinations which would have a substantial effect upon the practice in Massachusetts, but there may be some Massachusetts physicians here who can better answer that question.

Cathy Coleman (San Francisco, Calif.): I was in Massachusetts at that time and later spoke to Dr. *Hellman* at the Joint Center. There were about 185 patients referred to the Joint Center for Radiation Therapy for that procedure within 6 months to a year after the legislation was enacted. I find it disgusting that economic factors and benefits to the physicians would even be considered in individualized patient care for breast cancer.

Dr. Mehr (Marshfield, Wisc.): I wonder though if we pass broad legislation on informed consent, we're going to have a confused populace rather than an informed one. I think we must be prudent. It would be interesting as an internist if on a patient being admitted to the cardiac care unit I had to give him a piece of paper saying you could get IM pronestyl or you can get IV lidocaine or you can have digitalis, and this study says this, and have that patient sit there and read that for 10 min before I could do anything. I think this has some relevance, although there is a lot more emotion with regards to a woman's role. Last but not least, I think Mr. *Weinberg* said that we are a land of laws under law. Sometimes we might have too much law.

Front. Radiat. Ther. Onc., vol. 17, pp. 48–53 (Karger, Basel 1983)

Selection, Work-Up and Surgical Technique of Conservation Surgery and Axillary Dissection

Philip R. Westdahl

Children's Hospital of San Francisco, University of California, San Francisco, Calif., USA

Total mastectomy and axillary node dissection, the so-called modified radical mastectomy, has become the most widely used treatment of local-regional breast cancer at the present time. Unfortunately, 50% of patients with breast cancer already have distant metastases at the time of initial treatment. This, together with patint awareness of lesser surgical procedures and the demand for participation in decisions relating to their treatment, has led to a trend toward breast-conserving surgery and limited axillary node dissection followed by radiation therapy to the remaining breast and regional nodes if the latter are at risk of being involved. A review of the recent world literature tends to support the view that in selected patients, survival after breast-conserving surgery followed by adequate radiation is equivalent to radical and modified radical mastectomy at 5 years [3, 6, 9, 10] (table I) and in a few series at 10 years [1, 2, 7] (table II). Local recurrence appears to be higher for the lesser surgery-radiation group at 10 years (about 20%), but does not seem to have the same ominous prognostic imlications inasmuch as they can be treated by subsequent mastectomy without a significant decrease in survival. The answer may be that they are not true recurrences, but second primaries which have developed in the remaining breast tissue at risk.

Selection

All patients are not suitable candidates for breast-conserving treatment. The experience at the Curie Institute in Paris [2] has been that approximately 25% of their patients were suitable. The selection must be a

Table I. Milan Tumor Institute: 5-year evaluation (tumors <2 cm, no nodes palpable)

	Radical mastectomy	Quadrectomy and radiation
Cases, n	349	352
Survival		
Overall, %	90	90
NED, %	83	84
Stage I, %	89	87
Stage II, %	62	77
Local recurrence, n	3	1
Second primary, n		4
Distant METS, n	30	22

joint one between the patient, the surgeon and the radiotherapist based on many factors. Obviously, the patient must first of all have a tumor which meets the criteria to be outlined below. Assuming that she meets these criteria, she must have a desire to preserve her breast and understanding of the radiation therapy and its possible sequelae. It is for this reason that she should be seen by the radiotherapist prior to biopsy. Many patients prefer a mastectomy with the option of breast reconstruction. A well-performed total mastectomy and axillary dissection using a transverse incision, if feasible, and preserving skin without sacrifice of local cure is not the 'mutilating' procedure which it is so commonly claimed to be and lends itself to reconstruction with a very acceptable result. It is only after being fully apprised of the various alternatives that the patient can make her informed decision and this usually involves one or more lengthy discussions between the patient, the surgeon, the radiotherapist and usually the patient's husband.

There are several factors to be considered in the selection of patients for conservation treatment. *Tumor size* is important; obviously, the smaller the better. In the series of *Veronesi* et al [10] from the Milan Tumor Institute (table I), tumor size was selected as less than 2 cm and without palpable nodes. This series is perfectly matched, prospective and randomized. It includes 3,000 cases since 1960, of which 349 radical mastectomies and 352 quadrectomies and axillary node dissections are available

Table II. 10-year survival

Institution	Treatment	%	n
Columbia			
Stage I	radical mastectomy	76	455
Stage II	radical mastectomy	51	169
Memorial			
Stage I	radical mastectomy	76	166
Stage II	radical mastectomy	44	75
Marseilles			
Stage I	conservation and radiation	77	117
Stage II	conservation and radiation	60	117
Curie			
Stage I	conservation and radiation	75	135
Stage II	biopsy and radiation	38	34

for comparison at 5 years. The results are almost identical. With small tumors there is obviously better cosmesis as well as prolonged survival and minimal local recurrence.

Breast Size is also a factor in selection. If the breast is small in proportion to the size of the tumor, one cannot do even a limited resection without deforming the breast contour. In the case of a large, pendulous breast there is apt to be shrinkage following radiation leading to a poor cosmetic result. It is probably preferable in such patients to do a total mastectomy with a subsequent reconstruction on the side of the primary tumor and a reduction mammoplasty or subcutaneous mastectomy and reconstruction on the contralateral side.

Tumor location is a factor to be considered from the cosmetic aspect. Tumors in the upper and outer aspect of the breast lend themselves to the best results. On the other hand, tumors in the parasternal area where there is very little breast tissue are difficult to remove with an adequate margin and are prone to leave an obvious deformity.

There are several factors which render limited resection *unsuitable.*

One of these is *multicentricity,* particularly if the second tumor is in another quadrant where it cannot be removed through the same incision. Tumors with *poorly defined borders* such as diffuse lobular carcinoma are not suitable. Multicentric, occult, in situ carcinomas involve both of the above problems. *Subareolar tumors,* particularly with nipple retraction, require removal of the nipple-areolar complex and are therefore unsuitable from the cosmetic aspect. Finally, *large tumors,* greater than 5 cm, are unsuitable even in a large breast.

Work-Up

Every patient should have preoperative *mammograms.* A negative mammogram does not rule out carcinoma and should not deter biopsy of a suspicious abnormality on physical examination. The finding of a possible occult carcinoma in the same or contralateral breast is important for obvious reasons. A positive *bone scan* is very unlikely in tumors of the size and stage under consideration for limited surgery and radiation and is therefore not an essential part of the preoperative work up in these patients. A *fine needle biopsy* of a suspicious carcinoma is a simple office procedure and although it does not supplant a core needle biopsy or open biopsy for the unequivocal confirmation of cancer, it is of substantial help in the preoperative discussion which will enable the patient to take part in the final decision as to her treatment. It is accurate; false-positives are less than 1% and false-negatives are from 1 to 8% [8]. The combination of a suspicious finding on physical examination, mammograms and fine needle biopsy is 99% accurate in the diagnosis of breast cancer [8].

Technique

The technique of limited tumor resection varies from local resection with a narrow margin of breast tissue (lumpectomy, tylectomy, tumorectomy) to generous removal of the tumor and surrounding breast (quadrectomy, segmental resection, partial mastectomy). The latter technique may have a slight superiority relative to local recurrence as judged by the results of *Veronesi* et al. [9] and *Stehlin* et al. [9]. However, the cosmetic result may not be as satisfactory with tumors in the lower and medial aspect of the breast.

Axillary Dissection

It is important from the aspect of prognosis and possible need for adjuvant radiation or chemotherapy, to know the status of the axillary lymph nodes. It is also helpful to know at the time of surgery whether or not the nodes are involved. This can be determined by a 'touch prep' or by frozen section of any suspicious nodes. If either of these confirm the presence of metastases, a total axillary dissection should be performed. Postoperative radiation can then be limited to the supraclavicular nodes for lateral quadrant tumors and to supraclavicular and internal mammary nodes for medial quadrant tumors. There is some question of the efficacy of nodal radiation following adequate axillary dissection. The Milan Tumor Institute group has given up nodal radiation since 1976 in favor of adjuvant chemotherapy when axillary nodes contain metastases based on the known probability of concurrent distant metastases.

If the primary tumor is located in the upper outer quadrant, the incision for tumor resection can be extended into the axilla for node removal; for tumors in other locations, a separate, transverse axillary incision will provide adequate exposure. Because of the possibility of metastases to midaxillary nodes without involvement of the low axillary nodes, 21 % in one series [5], all nodes lateral and caudad to the lateral margin of the pectoralis minor muscle should be removed. If these are negative to touch prep or frozen section, removal of the higher nodes is probably not necessary and may avoid arm edema. Care should be taken to identify and protect the long thoracic and thoracodorsal nerves during the dissection.

Areas of Concern

(1) The firmness of breast and axillary tissue in some patients following limited surgery and radiation may mask local recurrence.

(2) There may be a potential, delayed, carcinogenic effect of radiation, particularly in young women. In most series in which radiation has been used as adjuvant postmastectomy therapy to the chest wall and regional nodes, the survival time has usually not been long enough to determine the possible carcinogenic effect on the surrounding tissues, particularly the contralateral breast. With prolonged survivals being reported in patients treated by limited surgery followed by irradiation, there is concern about the risk of carcinogenesis which may be small, but as yet has not been fully clarified [4].

References

1 Amalric, R.; Santamaria, F.; Robert, F.; Seigle, J.; Altschuler, C.; Kurtz, J.; Spitalier, J.; Brandone, H.; Ayme, Y.; Pollet, J.; Burmeister, R.; Abed, R.: Radiation therapy with or without primary limited surgery for operable breast cancer: a 20-year experience at the Marseilles Cancer Institute. Cancer *49:* 30–34 (1982).

2 Calle, R.; Pilleron, J.: Radiation therapy, with and without lumpectomy, for operable breast cancer: ten-year results. Breast *5:* 2–6 (1979).

3 Harris, J.; Botnick, L.; Bloomer, W.; Chaffey, J.; Hellman, S.: Primary radiation therapy for early breast cancer: the experience at the Joint Center for Radiation Therapy. Int. J. Radiat. Oncol. Biol. Phys. *7:* 1549–1552 (1981).

4 Harris, J.R.; Hellman, S.: Author's reply to letter to the editor from G. Kleinfeld re Possible hazards of radiation following local excision and radiation. Cancer *31:* 185–187 (1981).

5 Kitchen, P.; McLennan, R.; Mursell, A.: Node-positive breast cancer: a comparison of clinical and pathological findings and assessment of axillary clearance. Aust. N.Z. J. Surg. *50:* 580–583 (1980).

6 Montague, E.; Gutierrez, A.; Barker, J.; Tapley, N.; Fletcher, G.: Conservation surgery and irradiation for the treatment of favorable breast cancer. Cancer *43:* 1058–1061 (1979).

7 Mustakallio, S.: Conservative treatment of breast cancer – review of 25 years follow-up. Clin. Radiol. *23:* 110–116 (1972).

8 Russ, J.; Winchester, D.; Scanlon, E.; Christ, M.: Cytologic findings of aspiration of tumors of the breast. Surgery Gynec. Obstet. *146:* 407–411 (1978).

9 Stehlin, J., Jr.; Evans, R.; Gutierrez, A.; Cowles, J.; Ipolyi, P. de; Greeff, P.: Treatment of carcinoma of the breast. Surgery Gynec. Obstet. *149:* 911–922 (1979).

10 Veronesi, U.; Saccozzi, R.; Del Vecchio, M.; Banfi, A.; Clemente, C.; De Lena, M.; Gallus, G.; Greco, M.; Luini, A.; Marubini, F.; Muscolino, G.; Rilke, F.; Salvadori, B.; Zecchini, A.; Zucali, R.: Comparing radical mastectomy with quadrectomy, axillary dissection and radiotherapy with small cancers of the breast. New Engl. J. Med. *305:* 6–11 (1981).

P.R. Westdahl, MD, Children's Hospital of San Francisco, University of California, San Francisco, CA 94119 (USA)

Front. Radiat. Ther. Onc., vol. 17, pp. 54–59 (Karger, Basel, 1983)

Estrogen Receptors:
Significance and Current Status

Michael D. Lagios

Children's Hospital of San Francisco and University of California San Francisco, Calif.,
USA

Analysis of estrogen receptor (ER) – specifically the estradiol-17-beta-receptor – in human breast carcinoma, has provided a valuable insight into the biology of a significant human cancer and a mechanism for more rational choice of therapy in this disease.

ER are one of a large number of specific cellular proteins which are designed to bind a specific hormone and translocate the resulting hormone-receptor complex to the nucleus where a specific segment of the cell's DNA is activated. Most cells contain receptors for multiple hormones and both progesterone and prolactin receptors have been demonstrated in human breast cancers, but in our narrowed clinical perspective we are interested only in the estradiol-17-beta-receptor.

First identified in the rabbit myometrium, and since identified in almost every estrogen sensitive tissue, ER first came into clinical prominence as a means of predicting a more favorable response to adrenalectomy – a drastic endocrine ablative surgical procedure. ER, although still entirely valid in this situation, is presently more frequently used as a guide to prognosis.

The ER status of the patient's tumor can provide prognostic information regarding the likelihood of: short-term treatment failure, the disease-free interval, the overall survival, and survival after recurrence. Such a prognostic role for ER was first suggested by *Knight* et al. [10] who considered it as an independent prognostic factor for early recurrence. *Maynard* et al. [12] and, subsequently, *Bishop* et al. [2] from the Nottingham City Hospital noted that ER had no discriminant value for tumors at stage I, since all such lesions had a good prognosis, but that significant differences in disease-free interval were noted for stage II patients. Among

63 postmenopausal breast carcinoma patients at stage II, survival percentages for ER-positive versus ER-negative tumors were 89 versus 61% at 2 years, and 49 versus 15% at 3 years of follow-up. This survival reflects the results of simple mastectomy and limited node sampling but *no* adjuvant therapy. Many subsequent reports have confirmed these findings. *Rich* et al. [15] noted that 92% of ER-positive and 74% of ER-negative tumors remained disease-free over a 20-month follow-up period. *Gapinski and Donegan* [5] noted the corollary that 8% of ER-positive and 21% of ER-negative tumors recurred postmastectomy; *Samaan* et al. [16] confirmed increasing disease-free interval and survival in receptor-positive tumors, but only at stage II or higher. *Kinne* et al. [9] have shown that the poor prognosis associated with receptor-negative status is only valid for patients at stage II with 4 or more positive nodes. Controlling for tumor size, they noted no difference in recurrence rate or survival between ER-positive versus negative tumors at stage I or II with 3 or less nodes involved. This study also showed a significantly prolonged survival in receptor-positive as compared to receptor-negative tumors following the initial recurrence. Survival of ER-positive versus ER-negative tumors at 3 years of follow-up postrecurrence was 85 versus 50%, respectively.

A receptor-positive status, then, is statistically associated with a better prognosis in short-term follow-up, but also in overall survival and survival after recurrent disease has developed. Some early studies had suggested that a receptor-positive status also reflected a favorable response to chemotherapy but this has not been confirmed by subsequent studies. Nonetheless, receptor status appears to be a very useful adjunct to clinical management. Is it, however, an independent prognostic factor as *Knight* et al. [10] suggested, or does it reflect a more favorable tumor population which can be identified more conventionally?

The pioneering work of *Maynard* et al. [12] was also the first to identify a correlation between receptor status and degree of differentiation. There were significant differences in disease-free interval among receptor-positive and negative tumors of high grade, i.e., poorly differentiated (grade III), but no differences were identified among the better differentiated grade I and II tumors. *Rich* et al. [15], in the same year (1978), showed similarly an equal number of receptor-positive and negative tumors among histologic grade I and II carcinomas, but a much larger number of receptor-negative tumors at grade III, i.e., poorly differentiated. *Kern* [8] noted that receptor-negative tumors were associated with a lower nuclear grade, that is, more anaplastic (= de-differentiated) nuclei in fine needle aspirate

Table I. Relationship of receptor ER status to degree of differentiation

	ER +	ER –
Histologic grade	well – moderate (I–II)	Poor (III)
Nuclear grade	high (II–III)	low (I)
DNA ploidy	diploid	aneuploid
Growth rate (doubling time)	low	high
Host response	minimal	marked

analysis, as compared to receptor-positive tumors, which revealed higher nuclear grades and greater cohesiveness. *Antoniades and Spector* [1] noted that high nuclear grade tumors were receptor-positive in 93 % whereas low nuclear grade tumors (grade I) were receptor-negative in 67 % of cases. The latter authors also showed a correlation between histologic grade (= degree of differentiation) and receptor-positive status for better differentiated duct carcinomas particularly those with tubular features – a histologic hallmark of a highly differentiated duct carcinoma. *Fisher* et al. [4] and *Lessor* et al. [11] confirmed the association of receptor-positive status and low grade, that is, better differentiated carcinomas, and an inverse correlation with a number of prognostically unfavorable features: Low nuclear grade, i.e., anaplasia, high histologic grade (= poorly differentiated), prominent cellular host reaction, tumor necrosis and absence of elastosis.

Evaluation of histologic and nuclear grade is in practice, however, dependent on subjective evaluation and is subject to considerable observer bias and variation. Nonetheless, these subjectively determined features of a tumor – easily available to the practicing pathologist in an HE-stained slide – do correlate well with the level of in vitro thymidine labelling – an index of tumor doubling time, and DNA ploidy, an index of the degree of anaplasia of the tumor. These are objectively measurable features not subject to the same type of observer bias.

These observations are summarized in table I.

Well-differentiated tumors, characterized by high nuclear and low histologic grade, a slow doubling time in cell kinetic studies, a more normal diploid DNA content, and minimal cellular host reaction tend to be receptor-positive and are less likely to progress. Poorly differentiated tumors characterized by low nuclear and high histologic grade, a rapid doubling time, aneuploid DNA/cell content and marked host response tend to be receptor-negative [13, 14].

A positive receptor status will not be prognostically useful in histologically well-differentiated tumors, since disease is slowly progressive in these cases and no discriminate difference can be demonstrated. It is only in poorly differentiated breast carcinomas and breast carcinomas at stage II, those that have already metastasized to the axilla, that receptor status is prognostically useful. It would appear that receptor status is simply one of many features that reflect the degree of differentiation of the tumor and is not really independent of the general concept of grade. However, in the case of a poorly differentiated tumor at stage II it can provide very useful information which is not available to simple microscopic examination.

A few words about the tissue sample for receptor determination. First, the sample must contain tumor. It is an unfortunate practice in some hospitals to have a resident excise what he thinks is 'tumor', from a mastectomy specimen after an excision biopsy, without any histologic correlation or confirmation. As a result granulation tissue or in some cases normal breast is submitted for receptor determination and the patient consigned to a receptor-negative status and billed for a worthless laboratory procedure.

ER material is best reserved from a primary incision or excision biopsy as opposed to subsequent mastectomy. Such biopsy material provides identifiable tumor in a fresh state. An adequate sample of at least 500 mg should be quickly quenched in liquid nitrogen if available or frozen on dry ice, rather than allowed to sit for any length of time in the operating room or in the pathology laboratory, as some studies have shown a significant decrease in receptor activity even with the time required to complete the mastectomy [6].

We do not remove material from in situ carcinomas because there is no prognostic advantage to receptor status in such a patient and it is far more important to document an invasive focus in the biopsy which may have been limited to the fragments reserved for cytosol preparation and receptor study.

Receptor values do differ with the number of tumor cells sampled. Cellular tumors are more likely to have a receptor-positive value simply because more cells are available in the sample. The receptor is not contained within the desmoplastic host response or the cellular infiltrate of the tumor, as *Bennington* [this volume] will show. It is well worthwhile then to additionally sample a lymph node which has been replaced by metastatic carcinoma as this provides a much more homogeneous population of tumor cells than the primary site, particularly in cases of infiltrating lobular type. We have been able to demonstrate a tenfold difference in receptor values in such circumstances.

Axillary metastases can differ significantly from the primary tumor in receptor status, and in either direction. *Brennan* et al. [3] has shown up to a 34% variation in ER status between primary and axillary metastases. *Hoehn* et al.[7] note a 19% discrepancy. Therefore, metastases or local recurrences should never be assumed to be identical to the primary.

References

1 Antoniades, K.; Spector, H.: Correlation of estrogen receptor levels with histology and cytomorphology in human mammary cancer. Am. J. clin. Path. *71:* 497–503 (1979).

2 Bishop, H. M. et al.: Relationship of estrogen-receptor status to survival in breast cancer. Lancet *ii:* 283–284 (1979).

3 Brennan, M. J.; Donegan, W. L.; Appleby, D. E.: The variability of estrogen receptors in metastatic breast cancer. Am. J. Surg. *137:* 260–262 (1979).

4 Fisher, E. R. et al.: Correlation of estrogen receptor and pathologic characteristics of invasive breast cancer. Cancer *45:* 349–353 (1980).

5 Gapinski, P. V.; Donegan, W. L.: Estrogen receptors and breast cancer: prognostic and therapeutic implications. Surgery *88:* 386–393 (1980).

6 Hasson, J.; Luhan, P. A.; Kohl, M. W.: Comparison of estrogen receptor levels in breast cancer samples from mastectomy and frozen section specimens. Cancer *47:* 138–139 (1981).

7 Hoehn, J. L.; Plotka, E. D.; Dickson, K. B.: Comparison of estrogen receptor levels in primary and regional metastatic carcinoma of the breast. Ann. Surg. *190:* 69–71 (1979).

8 Kern, W. H.: Morphologic and clinical aspects of estrogen receptors in carcinoma of the breast. Surgery Gynec. Obstet. *148:* 240–242 (1979).

9 Kinne, D. W. et al.: Estrogen receptor protein in breast cancer as a predictor of recurrence. Cancer *47:* 2364–2367 (1981).

10 Knight, W. A. et al.: Estrogen receptor as an independent prognostic factor for early recurrence in breast cancer. Cancer Res. *37:* 4669–3671 (1977).

11 Lessor, M. L. et al.: Estrogen and progesterone receptors in breast carcinoma: correlations with epidemiology and pathology. Cancer *48:* 299–309 (1981).

12 Maynard, P. V. et al.: Estrogen receptor assay in primary breast cancer and early recurrence of the disease. Cancer Res. *38:* 4292–4295 (1978).

13 Meyer, J. S. et al.: Low incidence of estrogen receptor in breast carcinomas with rapid rates of cellular replication. Cancer *40:* 2290–2298 (1977).

14 Olszewski, W. et al.: Flow cytometry of breast carcinoma: I. Relation of DNA ploidy level to histology and estrogen receptor. Cancer *48:* 98–984 (1981).
15 Rich, M.A.; Furmanski, P.; Brooks, S.C.: Prognostic value of estrogen receptor determinations in patients with breast cancer. Cancer Res. *38:* 429–429B (1978).
16 Samaan, N.A. et al.: Estrogen receptor: a prognostic factor in breast cancer. Cancer *47:* 554–560 (1981).

M.D. Lagios, MD, Staff Pathologist, Children's Hospital of San Francisco,
San Francisco, CA 94119 (USA)

Front. Radiat. Ther. Onc., vol. 17, pp. 60–68 (Karger, Basel, 1983)

Immunoperoxidase Estrogen Receptor Assay for Human Breast Cancer

James L. Bennington

Department of Pathology, Children's Hospital of San Francisco, and West Coast Cancer Foundation, San Francisco, Calif., USA

Rationale for Use of the Estrogen Receptor Biochemical Assay

Breast cancer estrogen receptor (ER) content has proved to be an important guide to predicting the response to various forms of endocrine therapy for patients with metastatic disease [1, 6, 10]. Among unselected patients with disseminated carcinoma of the breast, approximately 30 % respond to endocrine therapy [5]. However, when selected according to tumor ER status, a high degree of accuracy can be obtained in predicting the response of individual patients to endocrine therapy, i. e., 55–>60 % for patients with ER-positive, but only 10 % for patients with ER-negative tumors (less than 3 fmol/mg of cytosol) [1, 11]. In general, the greater the concentration of ER found in tumor tissue, the more likely endocrine therapy will be effective [4].

Biochemical methods involving cytosol preparations from breast carcinoma homogenates have been used as a basis for establishing this relationship between ER status and tumor response to endocrine therapy. Currently, the two biochemical methods most widely used to measure tumor cytoplasmic ER content are the sucrose density gradient centrifugation assay and the dextran-coated charcoal assay [2, 21].

Deficiencies of the Biochemical Assay for ER Protein

Although well established as a standard for measuring breast carcinoma cytoplasmic ER content, the biochemical methods are subject to a number of practical and theoretical deficiencies [9]. The purpose of this

Table I. Major factors responsible for misclassification of ER status in human breast cancers

Improper handling and/or storage of tumor sample
Submission of specimen containing nontumor tissue
Submission of specimen, predominantly ER-negative, in a tumor composed of ER-positive and negative components
Dilution effect of stroma in sparsely cellular tumor
Blockage of receptor sites by patient's own estrogen in premenopausal women

Table II. Percent cancer cells in human breast carcinoma [from ref. 19]

Case number	Type	Tumor volume, mm³	Cancer cells, %
1	Infiltrating duct	1150	20.1
2	Infiltrating duct	382	42.8
3	Infiltrating duct	144	26.5
4	Infiltrating duct	268	3.9
5	Infiltrating duct	1023	6.6
6	Infiltrating duct	5960	11.2
7	Infiltrating duct	698	32.8
8	Infiltrating duct	1150	31.3
9	Infiltrating duct	268	10.1
10	Infiltrating duct	2142	39.3
11	Medullary	905	54.3
12	Medullary	449	76.4

review is to summarize the state of the art of immunohistochemical methods, particularly immunoperoxidase, as an alternative for assaying ER content in human breast cancers.

The biochemical ER assays are complex, time-consuming procedures requiring highly trained personnel, expensive equipment, and the use of radioisotopic tracers. As a result, it is not practical or economical for laboratories in small to medium size hospitals to perform these procedures. In addition, there are inherent problems with the biochemical ER assay that may result in failure to accurately predict tumor response to endocrine therapy, usually resulting in misclassification of ER-positive tumors as ER-negative. The factors responsible for the majority of false-negative classifications of tumor ER status are listed in table I.

While biochemical assays are routinely used to measure ER content per weight of protein in breast carcinomas, the extent to which the receptor protein being measured is representative of the tumor cannot be deter-

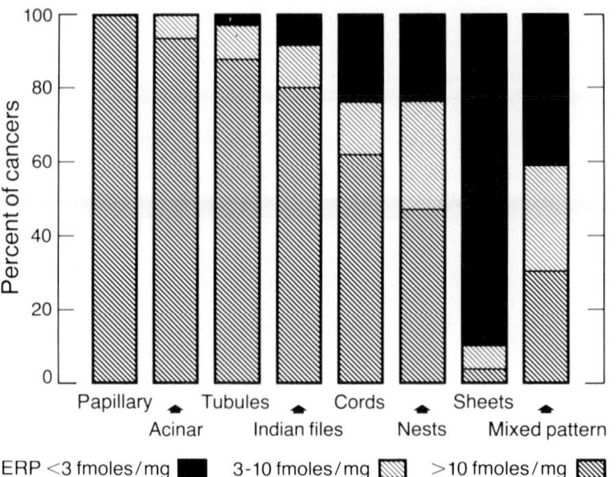

Fig. 1. Summary of the correlation of ER protein (ERP) and histologic patterns of breast cancers [from ref. 3].

mined with these procedures. Improper specimen handling or storage or both prior to performing the assay will result in loss or reduction in tumor receptor protein content. For reliable biochemical assay results, a specimen must be frozen immediately on dry ice or in liquid nitrogen. This offers limited opportunity for documenting the histology of the tissue submitted for assay. Submission of a specimen not representative of the tumor can produce a falsely low or negative ER value due to dilution of the tumor with normal tissue or in situ carcinoma low in ER protein. Correspondingly, dilution effect due to abundant stroma may produce false-negative results in ER-positive, but sparsely cellular tumors. This possibility is of considerable theoretical significance since invasive duct carcinomas of the breast are known to exhibit a wide range of cellularity. One study has shown a tenfold difference in the percent of total tumor volume made up of neoplastic cells in duct carcinomas of the breast [19] (table II).

Tumor ER content has been correlated with the histologic type and architectural pattern and degree of differentiation of invasive carcinomas of the breast [3, 16]. Among the histologic types of tumor, a high frequency of ER positivity is found among papillary carcinomas, tubular carcinomas, and infiltrating lobular carcinomas, while colloid and infiltrating duct carcinomas are of intermediate positivity and medullary carcinomas of low positivity (fig. 1). Certain histologic patterns show a high association with ER positivity including papillary, acinar, tubular and Indian file patterns

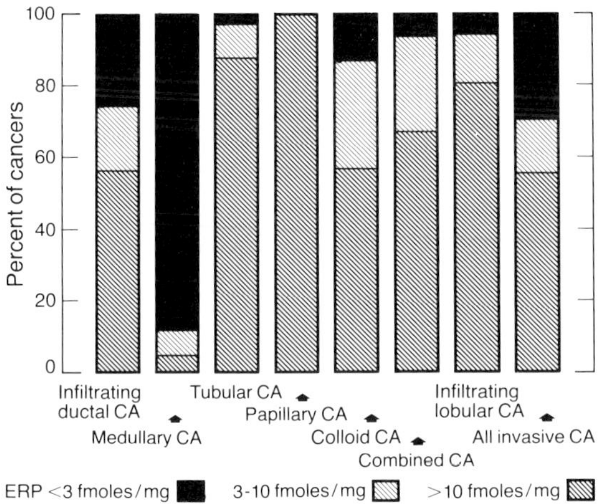

Fig. 2. Summary of the correlation of ERP and histologic types of breast cancers [from ref. 3].

while solid tumors show a high association with ER negativity (fig. 2). In general, well-differentiated breast carcinomas tend to be ER-positive (approximately 80 %) while poorly differentiated breast carcinomas have a low frequency of ER positivity (approximately 24 %) [3]. Heterogeneity of ER content within individual breast carcinomas is well documented [12]. This may, in part, be a manifestation of the variability of those morphologic features as they relate to ER content. In such tumors, false-negative results may be accounted for by the chance sampling of a predominantly ER-negative portion of an otherwise ER-positive tumor.

Finally, false-negative results may arise from assays of tumors from premenopausal patients. In such patients, tumor ER sites may be blocked by the patient's own estrogen. It is well documented that premenopausal women with plasma levels of estradiol less than 0.15 μM have low or undetectable amounts of ER in their tumors [18].

Immunohistochemical Assays for ER Content in Breast Carcinoma

Immunohistochemical procedures have been shown to hold considerable promise as alternative methods for detecting and quantifying ER content in human breast carcinomas. Immunofluorescent [7, 8, 13, 14] and immunoperoxidase methods [17, 20] have been adapted to this purpose.

Both methods overcome the major disadvantages of the biochemical cytoplasmic methods of ER assay discussed above. With both immunofluorescent and immunoperoxidase methods, processing is straightforward, requires less than 6 h to complete, does not require the use of radioisotopes and can be performed by a specially trained histotechnologist using standard laboratory equipment.

The immunoperoxidase method offers several advantages over the immunofluorescent method in that it does not depend on the use of a fluorescent microscope and does not require fresh tissue. The immunoperoxidase method is ideal for use on formalin-fixed and paraffin-embedded tissues and as such it is suitable for retrospective studies. The preparation provides a permanent record of the assay results.

Using immunohistochemical methods, ER is assayed indirectly by demonstrating intracellular estrogen bound to the receptor protein using labelled antibodies to estrogen. This procedure is performed on histologic sections and provides the means for direct correlation of tumor ER content with tumor morphology; a feature lacking in the biochemical assay. Slides of the tumor, after immunohistologic staining, can be used to quantify the percent of ER-positive tumor cells present and their distribution within the tumor. Because the sections are counterstained with conventional stains, they are also suitable for assessment of the presence of representative amounts of tumor in the sample, the degree of cellularity, grade, histologic type and architectural patterns of the invasive component of the tumor.

A relatively good correlation (89.4%) has been reported for the immunofluorescent and biochemical methods of ER measurement [15]. Similar results have been obtained in comparing immunoperoxidase and biochemical ER assays [17, 20] (fig. 3). With few exceptions, immunohistochemical measurements of ER are positive for all tumors found positive by biochemical assays. Moreover, they are positive for a significant number of tumors reported as negative by biochemical assay; biochemically negative tumors studied immunohistochemically may contain 10–20% ER-positive tumor cells [7, 12, 14, 15].

The finding that more tumors are classified as ER-positive with immunohistochemical than with biochemical assays may be accounted for by the following:

(1) With prompt formalin fixation of the tumor prior to immunoperoxidase staining, the ER complex is stabilized within the tumor, i.e., is not subject to subsequent loss or decay that may occur with improper handling of fresh specimens.

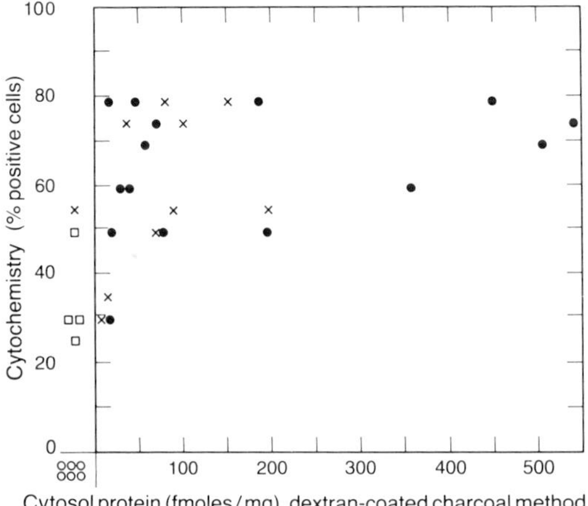

Fig. 3. Concentration and percentage positive cells (cytochemical method) for 35 breast carcinomas. Site of staining: ● = cytoplasmic and nuclear; × = cytoplasmic only; □ = nuclear only; ○ = negative [from ref. 20].

(2) With the immunoperoxidase method, tumors containing ER-positive cells are not incorrectly classified as ER-negative on the basis of inadequate sampling of the tumor or because the tumor is only sparsely cellular.

(3) The immunofluorescent and immunoperoxidase methods readily detect receptor protein in breast cancers of premenopausal women, while the biochemical assay may give false-negative results for such patients.

(4) Receptors located on the nucleus, when present, which are not detected by the biochemical assay, are frequently detected by the immuno fluorescent and immunoperoxidase methods [4, 12]. The significance of this difference; however, is not yet established.

Results obtained from immunofluorescent and immunoperoxidase assays indicate that it is unlikely that any breast carcinoma is composed entirely of ER-positive cells. On the other hand, breast carcinomas composed entirely of ER-negative cells are relatively common (15–25%) [8, 14, 17, 20] (table III).

Since the response to endocrine therapy seems to be proportional to the number of ER-positive cells in a tumor and since the purpose of the ER assay is to provide results that will form a basis for selecting those patients who will benefit from endocrine therapy, it is important that ER assays be

Table III. Mammary carcinomas according to percentages of receptor-positive cells in the cancer cell population [from ref. 8]

Positive cells	ER		Progesterone receptor	
%	number of tumors	percent	number of tumors	percent
>90	1	1.5	0	0
75–90	3	4.6	3	4.6
50–74	9	13.6	7	10.6
25–49	8	12	10	15.2
10–24	9	13.7	8	12
1–9	19	25.8	19	28.8
0	17	25.8	19	28.8
Total	66[1]	100	66[1]	100

[1] 63 primary and 3 metastatic carcinomas.

used that minimize false-negative results, and provide reliable estimates of the percentage of ER-positive cells for a given tumor.

With all of the practical and theoretical advantages of immunohistochemical methods for measuring ER protein in breast carcinoma, it is essential that prospective studies be carried out correlating the results of immunohistochemical ER assays with tumor response to endocrine therapy and that these results can be compared to those of conventional biochemical ER assays in terms of accuracy of predicting response to endocrine therapy.

Conclusions

The biochemical assay of ER protein in tumor cytosol has been established as a means to predict the response of patients with metastatic breast carcinoma to endocrine therapy. The biochemical assays have a number of practical and theoretical deficiences which favor immunohistochemical assay, particularly the immunoperoxidase method as an alternative for measuring ER content in human breast carcinomas. The major advantages of the immunoperoxidase method are as follows:

(1) The immunoperoxidase method is simple, requires less than 6 h to complete, does not require radioisotopes and can be performed by a specially trained histotechnologist using standard laboratory equipment.

(2) The immunoperoxidase procedure produces a color reaction at the binding site of ER protein within tumor cells providing a permanent record of the assay results.

(3) The immunoperoxidase method permits direct correlation of tumor ER content with tumor morphology which is important for proper interpretation of the results.

(4) With the immunoperoxidase method retrospective studies can be performed since the technique is suitable for formalin-fixed and paraffin-embedded tissues.

References

1   Allegra, J.C.; Lippman, M.E.; Thompson, E.B.; Simon, R.; Barlock, A.; Green, L.; Huff, K.K.; Do, H.M.; Aitken, S.C.; Warren, R.: Estrogen receptor status: an important variable in predicting response to endocrine therapy in metastatic breast cancer. Eur. J. Cancer *16:* 323–331 (1980).

2   Clark, J.H.; Peck, E.J.; Schrader, W.T.; et al.: Estrogen and progesterone receptors: methods for characterization and quantification. Methods Cancer Res. *12:* 367–417 (1976).

3   Fu, Y.S.; Maksem, J.A.; Hubay, C.A.; Temmim, L.; Reagan, J.W.: The relationship of breast cancer morphology and estrogen receptor protein status; in Fenoglio and Wolff, Progress in Surgical Pathology, vol.3, pp. 65–76 (Masson, New York 1981).

4   Heuson, J.C.; Longeval, E.; Mattheiem, W.H.; Deboel, M.C.; Sylvester, R.J.; Le Clercq, G.: Significance of quantitative assessment of estrogen receptor for endocrine therapy in advanced breast cancer. Cancer *39:* 1971–1977 (1977).

5   Howanitz, J.H.: Hormone receptors in breast cancer. Human Pathol. *12:* 1057–1059 (1981).

6   Jensen, E.V.; DeSombre, E.R.: The diagnostic implications of steroid binding in malignant tissues. Adv. Clin. Chem. *19:* 57–89 (1977).

7   Lee, S.H.: Cytochemical study of estrogen receptors in human mammary cancer. Am. J. Clin. Path. *70:* 197–203 (1978).

8   Lee, S.H.: Sex steroid hormone receptors in mammary cancer; in DeLellis, Diagnostic Immunohistochemistry, pp. 147–164 (Masson, New York 1981).

9   Maas, H.; Jonat, W.; Stolzenbach, G.; Trams, G.: The problem of non-responding estrogen receptor positive patients with advanced breast cancer. Cancer *46:* 2835–2837 (1980).

10 McGuire, W.L.; Carbone, P.P.; Volmer, E.,P.: Estrogen receptors in human breast cancer (Raven Press, New York 1975).

11 McGuire, W.L.: Steroid hormone receptors in breast cancer treatment strategy. Recent Prog. Horm. Res. *36:* 135–156 (1980).

12   Nenci, I.: Estrogen receptor cytochemistry in human breast cancer. Status and Prospects. Cancer *48:* 2674–2684 (1981).

13   Nenci, I.; Beccati, M. D.; Piffanelli, A.; Lanza, G.: Detection and dynamic localization of estrogen-receptor complexes in intact target cells by immunofluorescence technique. J. Steroid Biochem. *7:* 505–510 (1976).

14   Pertschuk, L. P.; Tobin, E. F.; Brigati, D. J.; Kim, D. S.; Bloom, N. D.; Gaetjens, E.; Berman, P. J.; Carter, A. C.; Degenshein, G. A.: Immunofluorescent detection of estrogen receptor in breast cancer. Comparison with dextran-coated charcoal and sucrose gradient assays. Cancer *41:* 907–411 (1978).

15   Pertschuk, L. P.: Detection of estrogen binding in human mammary carcinoma by immunofluorescence: a new technique utilizing the binding hormone in a polymerized state. Res. Commun. Chem. Pathol. Pharmacol. *14:* 771–774 (1976).

16   Silfverswärd, C.; Gustafsson, J. J.; Gustafsson, S. A.; Humla, S.; Nordenskjöld, B.; Wallgren, A.; Wrange, O.: Estrogen receptor concentration in 269 cases of histologically classified human breast cancer. Cancer *45:* 2001–2005 (1980).

17   Taylor, C. R.; Cooper, C. L.; Kurman, R. J.; Goebelsmann, U.; Markland, F. S., Jr.: Detection of estrogen receptor in breast and endometrial carcinoma by immunoperoxidase technique. Cancer *47:* 2634–2640 (1981).

18   Theve, N. O.; Carlström, K.; Gustafsson, J. A.; Gustafsson, S. A. Nordenskjöld, B.; Sköldefors, H.; Wrange, O.: Oestrogen receptors and peripheral serum levels of oestradiol-17 β in patients with mammary carcinoma. Eur. J. Cancer *14:* 1337–1340 (1978).

19   Underwood, J. C. E.: A morphometric analysis of human breast carcinoma. Br. J. Cancer *26:* 234–237 (1972).

20   Walker, R. A.; Cove, D. H.; Howell, A.: Histological detection of oestrogen receptors in human breast carcinomas. Lancet *i:* 171–173 (1980).

21   Witliff, J. L.: Steroid-binding proteins in normal and neoplastic mammary cells. Methods Cancer Res. *11:* 293–354 (1975).

J. L. Bennington, MD, Department of Pathology, Children's Hospital of San Francisco, 3700 California Street, San Francisco, CA 94118 (USA)

Front. Radiat. Ther. Onc., vol. 17, pp. 69–75 (Karger, Basel 1983)

Radiotherapy for Carcinoma of the Breast Instead of Mastectomy
An Update

Leonard R. Prosnitz[a], *Ira S. Goldenberg*[a], *Jay R. Harris*[b], *Samuel Hellman*[b], *Barbara F. Danoff*[c], *Simon Kramer*[c], *Paul E. Wallner*[d], *Luther W. Brady*[d]

[a] Departments of Therapeutic Radiology and Surgery, Yale University School of Medicine, New Haven, Conn., USA; [b] Joint Center for Radiation Therapy and Department of Radiation Therapy, Harvard University, Boston, Mass., USA; [c] Department of Radiation Therapy, Thomas Jefferson University Hospital, Philadelphia, Pa., USA; [d] Department of Radiation Therapy, Hahnemann Medical College, Philadelphia, Pa., USA

Radiation therapy as primary treatment for small carcinoma of the breast instead of mastectomy was introduced in Europe some 30 years ago [10]. Subsequently, thousands of patients, mostly in France, have been treated with radiation therapy [2, 3, 12], and large experience has also been acquired at the Princess Margaret Institute in Toronto, Canada [11]. These date will be described elsewhere in this symposium.

The first US reports did not appear until 1975 from the Yale [13] and Harvard [19] groups. Subsequently, many other US institutions have reported their experience [1, 9] and a large randomized prospective trial has been published from Milan [18]. All data suggest that this method of treatment is equivalent to mastectomy.

Shortly after the 1975 publications, the Yale and Harvard groups elected to pool their data along with the Jefferson and Hahnemann Medical Schools in Philadelphia because of a paucity of patients treated this way at any one institution, strong interest in the treatment of breast cancer in this manner at all four institutions, and similar treatment techniques being employed at all four institutions. The combined results have been previously published [14] and will be updated here.

Paralleling the upsurge of interest in primary radiotherapy instead of mastectomy, there has been a marked increase in the use of 'adjuvant' chemotherapy. The reasons for this are so well kown that they need not be repeated here. However, we are now faced with the complex problem of how to integrate surgical staging of the axilla, radiation and chemotherapy.

Rationale and Principles of Primary Radiation

Like surgery, radiotherapy is a local treatment, capable of achieving local control and curing the patient when there is no disease outside the local area. The ability of radiotherapy to be curative is well documented for diseases such as carcinoma of the larynx or cervical carcinoma [5]. It is rather surprising that there has been such resistance to the idea of radiation instead of surgery, as far as breast cancer is concerned. The radiobiological principles are well established – 4,500–5,000 rad (200 rad/day, 5 treatments/ week) are necessary for the control of microscopic or subclinical disease, with 6,000–7,000 rad or more necessary for palpable masses [6]. There are also numerous clinical studies demonstrating the ability of radiation to control microscopic breast cancer as well as clinically evident masses [5, 6]. Compared with surgery, radiotherapy has the obvious advantage of sparing the breast with all the attendant psychological benefits of avoiding mastectomy. The cosmetic appearance following radiation is generally much superior even when compared to mastectomy and subsequent reconstructive surgery.

Patient Selection

To ensure good results, not only in terms of disease control but also with good cosmesis, careful patient selection and attention to the details of treatment are necessary. The great majority of women with clinical stage I or II breast carcinoma are suitable for primary radiation with the following qualifications.

(1) The mass must be totally excised, although only a small margin (<1 cm) around the tumor is necessary. Therefore, the tumor: breast ratio must be small enough to permit excision without a significant deformity thereafter.

(2) Poorly defined primary tumors are not suitable because of the difficulty in totally excising them without removing a large part of the breast.

(3) Similarly, patients with several clinically evident masses within the breast are not suitable.

(4) Patients with grossly cystic breast disease in addition to the cancer should not be radiated if the cysts are large enough to be confusing at subsequent follow-up. However, some patients with cystic breast disease will have regression of the cysts following radiotherapy.

(5) Very obese women with very large pendulous breasts should not be treated by radiation because of the technical difficulties and the increased radiation reaction both

acutely, and more important, chronically. Such patients are usually better served by mastectomy and subsequent reconstruction.

Treatment Techniques

Surgical Aspects

An excisional biopsy should be done with only a small amount of surrounding normal breast. A 'quadrantectomy' is generally not necessary and will lead to a poor cosmetic result. It is, in fact, more difficult to reconstruct the breast after a partial than after a total mastectomy. If there are palpable axillary nodes, axillary dissection should be done, following the principle that all clinically evident tumor should be removed surgically. A separate transverse incision is usually employed for the axillary dissection.

Axillary surgery should also be done in the absence of palpable nodes if a decision regarding adjuvent chemotherapy is to be based on the result. There is a 25–45 % incidence of positive lymph nodes histologically when the axilla is clinically negative [4], the frequency depending on the size of the primary tumor. We favor a full dissection of the low and mid axilla, not a 'sampling', so that the axilla (except for the apex) can be excluded from the radiation field thereafter. Radiation therapy to the axilla following surgery greatly increases the frequency of arm edema.

Radiation Techniques

The appropriate doses of radiation have already been mentioned. We boost the primary site, limiting the volume to one third of the breast or less, using either an electron beam or iridium implantation and additional delivery of approximately 1,000–2,000 rad. The irradiated volume initially includes the entire breast and all the nodes, if there has been no axillary surgery. If axillary dissection has been done, the axilla is not irradiated, irrespective of the surgical findings (with certain rare exceptions). If the axilla is histologically negative, the other nodal groups are not irradiated except with a medial primary lesion. If the axilla is positive histologically, the internal mammary and the supraclavicular lymph nodes are treated.

Important technical factors include: limiting the fraction size to 200 rad/day; use of wedge filters; avoidance of bolus, and avoidance of overlap at field margins. The technical aspects of treatment have been detailed in several publications [8, 14].

Results of Primary Radiation Therapy

293 patients have now been treated in this cooperative four institutional trial, and followed for a minimum of 2 years and a maximum of 12. 36 of these patients have had axillary surgical procedures and 34 patients including 23 of the 36 have had subsequent adjuvant chemotherapy. These patients are all in the group with the shortest follow-up so their survival does not differ as yet from the overall patient group. They are therefore not further separated in the data analysis.

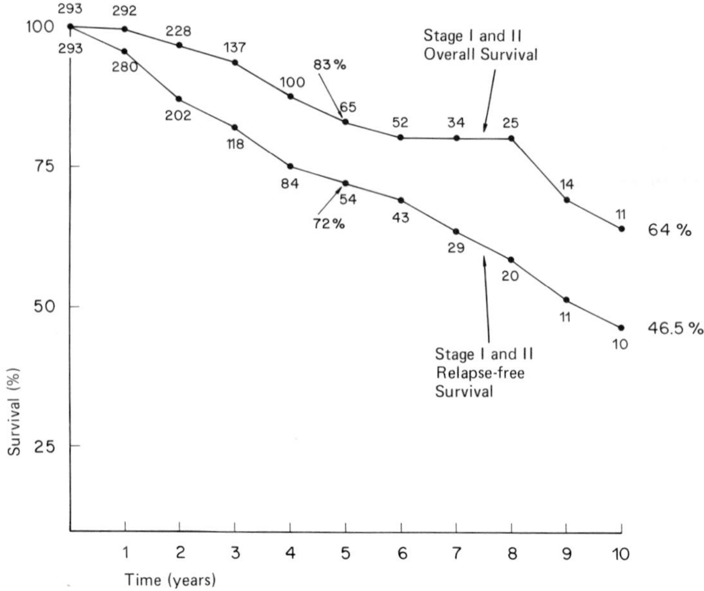

Fig. 1. Overall survival and relapse-free survival of 293 patients with breast cancer treated primarily with radiation.

Survival and relapse-free survival in the 293 patients are shown in figure 1. At 5 and 10 years, 80 and 64 % of patients are alive, with 72 and 46 % alive and free of disease. The incidence of local control is 92 %. There have been 23 local recurrences, 19 in the breast, 2 in the breast and regional nodes, and 2 in the lymph nodes only. Approximately one half of these patients are alive and free of disease following surgical resection, usually mastectomy.

Complications of radiation have occurred in 40 patients, none fatal and mostly not serious. The most frequent was rib fracture in 11 patients, apparently related to a fractionation scheme earlier in the study of 250 rad/ day and only seen once with a 200-rad/day treatment plan. Radiation pneumonitis occurred in 7 patients with residual lung damage in 1 patient. 4 patients had a brachial plexus injury (sensory only), 5 had permanent restriction of arm motion, 2 had arm edema, 8 had excessive fibrosis and the others a variety of problems that were self limited and possibly not even radiation related.

Table I. Primary radiotherapy trials

Reference	Number of patients	Clinical stage	Survival, %			Local recurrences %
			5 years	relapse free	10 years	
2	1,099	I and II	72	68	65	10
3	120	I	85 +	85	75 +	9
9	169	I and II	86 +	86	–	4
11	203	I and II	86	80	72	8
12	134	I and II	82	77	–	7
18	352	I	89	83	–	–
20	293	I and II	85	74	64	8

Second malignancies were not observed outside the breast. A radiation-induced cancer in the treated breast would be indistinguishable from local recurrence. Since the frequency of local recurrence appears comparable to that seen following mastectomy, it is very unlikely that a significant number of radiation-induced breast carcinomas occurs.

Cosmetic results have been generally very satisfactory but we are unable to quantify these further at the present time.

Discussion

The results obtained in non-randomized studies from single institutions are always difficult to compare to other studies. Nevertheless there has been fairly remarkable agreement in the results of primary radiation at major centers around the world. Table I lists some of the more important studies. It includes the randomized trial from Milan, with 700 patients showing no difference in survival or relapse-free survival between the irradiated patients and those undergoing mastectomy [18]. This trial is also important because all patients had axillary dissections and all node-positive patients received adjuvant chemotherapy. There was no suggestion that radiation interfered with the ability to give chemotherapy or adversely influenced the survival of node-positive patients receiving chemotherapy. Comparison of the results of primary irradiation with some of the major published surgical series [7, 15, 17] also strongly suggests that there are no differences in survival or local recurrence between patients having a mastectomy and those treated with primary irradiation.

Conclusion

Evidence has now accumulated from a large number of centers in many parts of the world showing that survival and relapse-free survival following primary radiotherapy for breast carcinoma are virtually identical to that seen when mastectomy is used as the primary method of treatment. Longer follow-up on some of the irradiated patients is clearly desirable. Nevertheless, there are enough data available concerning primary radiotherapy that surgeons and other physicians caring for breast cancer patients have an obligation to make the patient aware that alternatives to mastectomy do exist. As women become aware of other treatment options besides mastectomy, they may seek medical attention sooner and be diagnosed with smaller primary lesions with a real resulting improvement in cure rates.

References

1   Alpert, S.; Ghossein, N. A.; Stacey, P. et al.: Primary management of operable breast cancer by minimal surgery and radiotherapy. Cancer *42:* 2054–2058 (1978).
2   Amalric R.; Santamaria, F.; Robert, F. et al.: Radiation therapy with or without primary limited surgery for operable breast cancer: a 20 year experience at the Marseilles Cancer Institute. Cancer *49:* 30–34 (1982).
3   Calle, R.; Pilleron, J. P.; Schlienger, P.; Vilcoq, J. R.: Conservative management of operable breast cancer: 10 years experience at the Foundation Curie. Cancer *42:* 2045–2053 (1978).
4   Fisher, B.; Wolmark, N.; Bauer, M. et al.: The accuracy of clinical nodal staging and of limited axillary dissection as a determinant of histologic nodal status in carcinoma of the breast. Surgery Gynec. Obstet. *152:* 765–772 (1981).
5   Fletcher, G. H.: Textbook of radiotherapy; 3rd ed. (Lea & Febiger, Philadelphia 1980).
6   Fletcher, G. H.: Clinical dose response curves of human malignant epithelial tumors. Br. J. Radiol. *46:* 1–12 (1973).
7   Handley, R. S.: The conservative radical mastectomy of Patey: 10 year results in 425 patients. Breast *2:* 16–19 (1976).
8   Levene, M. B.; Harris, J. R.; Hellman, S.: Treatment of carcinoma of the breast with radiation therapy. Cancer *39:* 2840–2845 (1977).
9   Montague, E. D.; Gutierrez, A. E.; Barker, J. L. et al.: Conservation surgery and irradiation for the treatment of favorable breast cancer. Cancer *43:* 1058–1061 (1979).

10   Mustakallio, S.: Treatment of breast cancer by tumor extirpation and roentgen therapy instead of radical operation. J. Fac. Radiol. *6:* 23–26 (1954).

11   Peters, M. V.: Wedge resection with or without radiation in early breast cancer. Int. J. Radiat. Oncol. Biol. Phys. *2:* 1151–1156 (1977).

12   Pierquin, B.; Owen, R.; Maylin, C. et al.: Radical radiation therapy in breast cancer. Int. J. Radiat. Oncol. Biol. Phys. *6:* 17–24 (1980).

13   Prosnitz, L.R.; Goldenberg, I.S.: Radiation therapy as primary treatment for early stage carcinoma of the breast. Cancer *35:* 1587–1596 (1975).

14   Prosnitz, L.R.; Goldenberg, I.S.; Packard R.A. et al.: Radiation therapy as initial treatment in early stage cancer of the breast without mastectomy. Cancer *39:* 917–923 (1977).

15   Robinson, G.N.; Van Heerden, J.A.; Payne, W.S. et al.: The primary surgical treatment of carcinoma of the breast: a changing trend to a modified radical mastectomy. Mayo Clin. Proc. *51:* 433–442 (1976).

16   Schottenfeld, D.; Nash, A.G.; Robbins, G.F.; Beattie, E.J.: Ten year results of the treatment of primary operable breast cancer. Cancer *38:* 1001–1007 (1976).

17   Valagussa, P.; Bonadonna, G.; Veronesi, U.: Patterns of relapse and survival following radical mastectomy. Cancer *41:* 1170–1178 (1978).

18   Veronesi, U.; Saccozzi, R.; Del Vecchio, M. et al.: Comparing radical mastectomy with quadrantectomy, axillary dissection and radiotherapy in patients with small cancers of the breast. New Engl. J. Med. *305:* 6–11 (1981).

19   Webber, E.; Hellman, S.: Radiation as primary treatment for local control of breast carcinoma. J. Am. med. Ass. *234:* 608–611 (1975).

20   Prosnitz, L.R.; Goldenberg, I.S.; Harris, J.R. et al.: Primary radiotherapy for stage I and II breast cancer: A follow-up report from four East Coast University hospitals. Int. J. Radiat. Oncol. Biol. Phys. *6:* 1339–1340 (1980).

L.R Prosnitz, MD, Departments of Therapeutic Radiology and Surgery, Yale University, School of Medicine, New Haven, CT 06510 (USA)

Front. Radiat. Ther. Onc., vol. 17, pp. 76–83 (Karger, Basel 1983)

Conservation Surgery and Irradiation in the Treatment of Breast Cancer [1]

E. D. Montague[a], *S. R. Schell*[a], *M. D. Romsdahl*[b], *F. C. Ames*[b]

[a] Divison of Radiotherapy and [b] Department of Surgery, University of Texas,
M.D. Anderson Hospital and Tumor Institute at Houston, Houston, Tex., USA

The treatment of breast cancer has undergone substantial changes in the past 20 years. Conventional radical mastectomy has been partly replaced by the more conservative modified radical, while the extended radical mastectomy has been, by and large, abandoned. Radiation therapy has gained favor as a therapeutic modality for patients with clinically favorable cancer who desire conservation of the breast. This paper reviews the results of radiation treatment making particular reference to the complications and the incidences of second primaries either in the breast or different sites.

Materials

Table I shows the staging distribution of 263 patients treated with conservation surgery and irradiation. All patients had biopsy-proved breast cancer without distant metastases; 31 had noninvasive and 232 had invasive cancer. Prior to 1974, involvement of the axilla was established only by clinical examination; a dissection of the lateral axilla has been performed since 1974, so that histologic staging is available for some patients. Excision was done in 123 patients prior to referral and in 140 patients at The University of Texas M.D. Anderson Hospital and Tumor Institute at Houston (UT MDAH). Initially, patients were referred for radiotherapy following excision of a primary tumor because of patient refusal to undergo mastectomy, poor medical condition precluding anesthesia and surgery, or peripherally placed primaries in either the inframammary sulcus or the parasternal area. Recently, patients were selected for conservative treatment by the surgeon and radiotherapist. The options are discussed with each patient.

[1] This investigation was supported in part by grand No. CA06294, awarded by the National Cancer Institute and the Departments of Health and Human Services.

Table I. Clinical stage of patients treated with conservation sugery and irradiation (1955–1979; analysis January 1982)

Noninvasive	31
Stage I (T_1N_0)	
Clinically negative axilla	76
Histologically negative axilla	35
Stage II (T_1N_1, T_2N_0)	
Clinically negative	45
Histologically negative	19
Clinically positive	24
Histologically positive	33

Table II. Areas irradiated[1] following excision of a carcinoma and axillary dissection [from ref. 3]

	Radiotherapy fields	
Histology of nodes	outer quadrant primary	central or inner quadrant primary
–	breast	breast internal mammary chain
+	breast internal mammary chain supraclavicular	breast internal mammary chain supraclavicular

[1] Without axillary dissection and excluding minimal breast cancer (in situ lobular, intraductal noninvasive, or invasive mass < 5 mm in diameter), irradiation is delivered to the breast, axilla, internal mammary chain, and supraclavicular nodes.

Irradiation of the breast has been given with ^{60}Co through medial and lateral tangential portals; the entire breast and chest wall were irradiated generally without the use of bolus and during the last 7 years, using open and wedge-filtered fields when the tumor is far away from the nipple, for a total tumor dose of 5,000 rad in 5 weeks plus an additional 1,000 rad TD to the site of the excised tumor usually with electrons. During the last 5 years, some patients with clear margins did not receive a boost. Patients with noninvasive cancer had only the breast irradiated. For those without an axillary dissection, a 5,000 rad tumor dose was delivered to the axilla and to the supraclavicular area through the anterior supraclavicular-axillary field and the posterior axillary field, opposing the low and central axilla. The internal mammary nodes were irradiated through a direct field for 4,500 rad tumor dose in 5 weeks [2]. In recent years, photons and electrons have been mixed, particularly for treating the internal mammary and the supraclavicular nodes. Following either a complete axillary dissection or, what is much preferred, a dissection of the lateral axilla, the areas irradiated depend on the histologic axillary status and the site of the primary tumor in the breast (table II) [3].

Results

The rate of failure was 8.1% in 123 patients in whom the excision had been done prior to referral, and only 2.9% in 140 patients having the excision at UT MDAH [4]. The difference is undoubtedly related to incomplete excision performed, in many instances, by surgeons who were not aware that excision biopsy would be the only surgical procedure. This higher failure rate has led, for patients who had prior excision, to a re-excision whenever possible of the primary site, in addition to a dissection of the lateral axilla. This is done in an effort to limit the radiation dose to 5,000 rad TD for subclinical disease rather than the higher radiation dose that would be required to treat possible gross disease. If the re-excision is negative for carcinoma, no boost is delivered.

As has been reported previously, the survival rates of those patients treated with conservation surgery and irradiation are comparable, stage by stage, to the survival rates of patients treated with radical mastectomy [5].

Cosmetic Results

The cosmetic results vary depending on both the surgical and the radiation technique. They are good to excellent in 75% of patients. Elliptical incisions are suggested for tumor excision in the upper half of the breast, and radial incisions for the lower half. In addition, the axillary dissection incision should be a separate one even when the primary tumor is in the upper outer quadrant, unless the tumor is in the tail of the breast. The radiotherapist must avoid junction overlaps by carefully setting up fields, and by reducing the volume to be irradiated. For example, if a lateral axillary dissection is done, and the nodes are either negative or positive but less than 2 cm in size, only the axillary apex needs irradiation.

A previous report on late complications from MDAH has described the long-term complications from protracted irradiation for far advanced cancer of the breast showing that long follow-up is necessary before final evaluation can be made [7]. However, if patients treated with 5,000 rad in 5 weeks (25 fractions) have a good cosmetic result at 5 years, they are likely to

Table III. Complications of conservation surgery and irradiation for clinically favorable breast cancer in 263 patients (1955–1979; analysis 1982)

Complication	%	patients, n
Symptomatic pneumonitis		
^{60}Co	9	16/178
^{60}Co + electrons	2	2/85
Rib fracture	1.5	4
Severe fibrosis at field junctions	14	36
Severe fibrosis entire breast	4	10
Breast necrosis	0.4	1[1]
Fat necrosis	0.8	2[2]
Pleural effusion, transient	0.8	2
Brachial plexopathy	1	3[3]
Arm edema	7	6/87[4]
Breast edema	22	19/87[5]

[1] Patient had scleroderma.

[2] Tender mass in irradiated field, biopsied.

[3] One minimal transient sensory change. One moderate stable sensory loss. One severe sensory and motor loss, only patient receiving adjuvant chemotherapy (vincristine, adriamycin, cytoxan + methotrexate and 5-FU).

[4] Occurred only after axillary dissection; 4 after complete dissection, and 2 after low dissection.

[5] Occurred only after axillary dissection, either complete or partial.

remain good, whereas if there is early fibrosis of the breast and soft tissues, there can be severe complications in 10–15 years.

Pneumonitis

Asymptomatic apical fibrosis, reported previously in almost every patient, and 10% incidence of symptomatic pneumonitis have been significantly reduced with the use of a mixture of photons and electrons for the supraclavicular and the internal mammary chain field. As seen in table III, only 2 of 85 patients treated with ^{60}Co and electrons in these two fields have suffered symptomatic pneumonitis, and both of these patients had a wide tangential field separation necessitated by a long scar that required irradiation in the lateral chest wall.

Fibrosis

Because the technique used for the more advanced local and regional disease was carried over into the patients treated for early and clinically favorable disease, patients who were treated in the earlier years had their junction lines treated twice in order to avoid a cold area, particularly when the tumor bed was split by the junction.

Fat Necrosis

Fat necrosis has occurred as a slightly tender subcutaneous mass in the irradiated field. Biopsy is always indicated.

Necrosis

Patients with collagen diseases treated with irradiation show an excessive incidence of complications. The 1 patient in this series who developed necrosis after 5,000 rad in 5 weeks had generalized scleroderma. The necrosis has been excised and the patient continues to be well 4 years after irradiation; however, she has considerable fibrosis of the entire treated area.

Pleural Effusion

The 2 patients who developed transient pleural effusion within 4 months of the radiation therapy had wide tangential field separation, so that a large volume of pleural surface was irradiated by the tangential fields. 1 patient remains well 5 years after treatment; the other developed bilateral pleural effusion, positive for tumor, 6 months after unilateral pleural effusion that was negative for cancer cells. It is possible that she had a unilateral pleural effusion secondary to tumor, but this was never proved.

Brachial Plexopathy

A report in preparation [1] indicates that the overall incidence of brachial plexopathy in patients with breast cancer of all stages treated with radiation in UT MDAH is approximately 0.4%, and that brachial plexopathy increases when a boost of more than 1,000 rad given dose in 5 days is delivered to a limited field in the supraclavicular area, or through appositional fields in the axilla. 2 of 3 patients listed in table III were treated to 5,000 rad given dose in 25 fractions to the anterior supraclavicular-axillary portal, and 5,000 rad tumor dose to the midaxilla by means of a posterior axillary field, in addition to a boost of 1,500 rad tumor dose with 11-MeV electrons to a clinically positive axillary node through an appositional field. 1 patient has minimal transient sensory change, and another has had a stable sensory loss for 8 years. A third patient, who has sensory and motor loss, was given no boost to either the axilla or supraclavicular area, the latter portal receiving 4,000 rad given dose in 20 fractions with ^{60}Co and an additional 1,000 rad given dose with 6-MeV electrons. Following radiation therapy, however, this patient was treated with vincristine, adriamycin and cyclophosphamide (Cytoxan), followed by methotrexate and 5-fluorouracil (5-FU) for 2 years, and developed brachial plexopathy in the second year.

Edema

In 1974, when it was decided that histologic evaluation of the axilla was necessary, the first 9 patients had a complete axillary dissection. 6 of these patients developed significant arm edema, was well as a retrograde breast edema that lasted for 3–4 years. Following the dissection, breast edema can occur prior to the irradiation and has clinical manifestations similar to inflammatory carcinoma with erythema, peau d'orange, and ridging. Radiation therapy does not appear to make the edema worse, but the skin thickening on follow-up xeromammograms can be confused with recurrent disease, so that all clinicians should be made aware of the problem. Following this high incidence of complications with a complete axillary dissection, it was decided to perform only a dissection lateral to the pectoralis minor; since this change, 2 patients have had transient upper arm edema, but breast edema has occurred in some patients.

Incidence of Other Primary Cancer

Table IV is an analysis of all patients with stages I and II breast cancer treated at UT MDAH, 6% of whom have developed a cancer in the remaining breast [6]. When the incidence of the opposite breast malignancy is studied as a function of the treatment to the first breast, it is seen that patients who were treated with combined surgery and radiation therapy for the first treatment have no greater incidence of second breast cancer (3.4%) than patients whose first breast cancer was treated with surgery alone (7.3%). These data were accumulated from patients treated between 1948 and 1976, based on a 5-year follow-up on patients; at that time only 98 patients treated with excision and irradiation had been accumulated. There is no evidence, at least in this patient group, that the radiation therapy used in the treatment of a first breast cancer is conducive to the development of a second breast cancer.

Table V shows the incidence of other primary tumors in the patients with breast cancer treated from 1948 through 1978 at UT MDAH. There is

Table IV. Bilateral breast cancer: consecutive presentation in stages I and II (T_1N_0, T_2N_1) (1948–1976; analysis January 1981): incidence of second breast cancer correlated with the treatment of the first breast [from ref. 6]

Treatement		Number of patients developing second breast primary (%)		
Surgery only		30/409	(7.3)	
Peripheral lymphatic irradiation		27/553	(4.9)	
Peripheral lymphatic + electron beam chest wall irradiation		7/321	(2.2)	
Irradiation of chest wall with tangential portals	simple mastectomy	5/228	(2.2)	57/1,673 (3.4)
	wedge excision	0/98	–	
	pre-op and radical mastectomy	18/473	(3.8)	

Table V. Incidence of multiple primary cancers excluding breast in patients with breast cancer treated with surgery alone or surgery and irradiation (1948–1978; analysis November 1980) [from ref. 5]

	Surgery alone	Surgery and irradiation
Total number of patients	700	3,713
Number of patients developing second primary tumors after treatment to breast	9 (1.3) *	75 (2.0) *

* $p = 0.19$.

no statistical difference between the patients treated with surgery alone and those treated with combined surgery and irradiation. The most common second-primary malignancies, excluding skin cancers, in both groups were gynecological and colorectal cancers, and in the last 4 years under review, an increasing incidence of lung cancer.

Discussion

Although the complications secondary to conservative surgery and irradiation are not fully known, since not enough patients have yet been followed for over 10 years, the sequelae will be fewer than the late complications of high-dose irradiation for far-advanced local-regional disease. The cosmetic results depend on the cooperative efforts of the surgeon and the radiotherapist in selecting suitable patients and in treatment techniques (surgery and radiation).

There is no evidence in this series of patients of increased cancer in the remaining breast, or in any site relative to the use of radiation in the treatment of the first breast.

References

1   Fields, R.; Glass, P.; Spanos, W.J., Jr.; Montague, E.D.: Brachial plexopathy after radiation therapy for treatment of breast cancer (in preparation).
2   Fletcher, G.H.: Textbook of radiotherapy; 3rd ed. (Lea & Febiger, Philadelphia 1980).
3   Montague, E.D.; Gutierrez, A.E.; Barker, J.L.; Tapley, N. duV.; Fletcher, G.H.: Conservation surgery and irradiation for the treatment of favorable breast cancer. Cancer 43: 1058–1061 (1979).
4   Montague, E.D.; Paulus, D.D.; Schell, S.R.: Selection and follow-up of patients for conservation surgery and irradiation. Front. Radiat. Ther. Onc. 17: 124–130 (Karger, Basel 1983).
5   Montague, E.D.; Spanos, W.J., Jr.; Ames, F.; Romsdahl, M.; Schell, S.R.; Fletcher, G.H.; Oswald, M.J.: Conservation surgery and irradiation for the treatment of clinically favorable breast cancer; in McLelland, Feig, Breast carcinoma: current diagnosis and treatment (Masson, Paris 1982).
6   Schell, S.R.; Montague, E.D.; Spanos, W.J, Jr.; Tapley, N. duV.; Fletcher, G.H.; Oswald, M.J.: Bilateral breast cancer in patients with initial stage I and II disease. Cancer (in preparation, 1982).
7   Spanos, W.J., Jr.; Montague, E.D.; Fletcher, G.H.: Late complications of radiation only for advanced breast cancer. Int. J. Radiat. Oncol. Biol. Phys. 6: 1473–1476 (1980).

Prof. E.D. Montague, MD, Division of Radiotherapy, University of Texas, M.D. Anderson Hospital and Tumor Institute at Houston, Houston, TX 77030 (USA)

Front. Radiat. Ther. Onc., vol. 17, pp. 84–90 (Karger, Basel 1983)

Results of Salvage Surgery for Local Failure following Conservative Therapy of Operable Breast Cancer

John M. Kurtz[a], *Jean-Maurice Spitalier*[b], *Robert Amalric*[b]

[a] Swedish Hospital Tumor Institute, Seattle, Wash., USA;
[b] Institut J. Paoli-I. Calmettes, Marseilles, France

Local recurrence following radical surgery conveys a grave prognosis to the breast cancer victim. Although local failure sometimes occurs in a setting of obvious disease dissemination, even women who have apparently isolated chest wall or nodal recurrences after mastectomy have only a 20–30% 5-year survival [2, 5] and a 10-year survival of less than 10%, implying that such patients are only rarely curable by further therapy. This conclusion does not necessarily apply, however, to patients who have recurrences in the intact breast or axilla following conservation therapy with radiation. Although there are no articles in the literature devoted exclusively to this issue, several reports from European centers provide data to suggest that local failure after limited surgery and irradiation is treatable by further surgery with rather satisfactory results [4, 6, 8, 9]. This paper will examine in some detail the extensive experience with such salvage surgery at the Cancer Institute in Marseilles, and then tabulate similar data from other sources in the literature, primarily from France.

Materials and Methods

Between June 1960 and December 1981, 3,786 operable breast cancers (T1–3, NO–1) were treated by curative radiation therapy with or without primary limited surgery, the latter consisting mostly of lumpectomy or wedge excision, and only most recently including limited axillary dissection in selected patients. This study is limited to those 704 patients treated prior to December 1971, thus having a minimum of 10 years follow-up. This represents an unselected series of breast cancer of all operable stages. Treatment policies and techniques have previously been described [1]. Tumor excision was performed prior to radiotherapy in 283 T1 and T2 lesions, having minimal or no adenopathy and no clinical signs of rapid growth.

The remaining 421, generally more advanced cases, were treated with curative radiotherapy following biopsy, without tumor excision. Long-term survival rates have previously been published [1]. Patients were submitted to a secondary operation, usually a radical mastectomy, if they were suspected of having local or regional tumor persistence or recurrence and had no evidence of distant metastatic disease at the time.

Results

With follow-up ranging from 10 to 21 years, a total of 227 local-regional failures were documented, 57 in patients treated by excision and radiotherapy, and 170 after radiotherapy without excision. Of these 227 patients, 48 (21%) were unable to have a salvage operation, largely due to the presence of distant metastases or to the extent of the local recurrence. Operability was somewhat higher in the early-stage patients; 90% of the 67 failures among the initially stage I (T1–2, NO) cases were operable, whereas only 74% of the 160 initial stage II and III failures could have secondary operations. Parenthetically, an additional 56 patients had a secondary operation for suspected recurrence, but the surgical specimen was histologically negative. These patients are not the object of further consideration.

Although current practice in Marseilles now favors the modified radical mastectomy, in the time frame of this study, 117 (65%) of the salvage operations were classical Halsted radical mastectomies, with the modified Patey mastectomy employed in only 30 instances (17%), simple mastectomy in 11 (6%), and a conservative secondary operation (wedge resection and/or axillary dissection) in 21 cases (12%). For those patients subjected to radical secondary operations, morbidity largely involved a significant delay in wound healing plus a higher incidence of arm edema (29%) than with primary radical mastectomy. Only rarely was this disabling, however. There was less morbidity with the Patey than with the Halsted operation, and the morbidity of the conservative salvage operations was minimal.

The remainder of this analysis is devoted to 147 histologically proven local-regional failures operated prior to January 1977, thus having a minimum of 5 years follow-up after the salvage operation. At surgery, 69 patients (47%) were found to have positive axillary nodes, including 14/45 (31%) of initial stage I (T1–2, NO), 30/61 (49%) of initial stage II (T1–2, N1) and 25/41 (61%) of initial stage III (T3, NO–1) cases. 5 years after

Table I. 5-year survival after salvage surgery

Original clinical stage	N +		N −		Total	
	n	%	n	%	n	%
Stage I (T1–2, N0)	5/14	36	22/31	71	27/45	60
Stage II (T1–2, N1)	11/30	37	23/31	74	34/61	56
Stage III (T3, N0–1)	6/25	24	8/16	50	14/41	34
Overall	22/69	32	53/78	68	75/147	51

N + = Proven axillary metastases at time of secondary operation.

Table II. Disease-free survival at 10 years after *primary* therapy

Original clinical stage	Salvage surgery for proven local-regional failure		Not requiring salvage surgery for failure[1]	
	n	%	n	%
Stage I (T1–2, N0)	42/60	70	157/225	70
Stage II (T1–2, N1)	37/75	49	94/172	55
Stage III (T3, N0–1)	13/44	30	31/80	39

[1] Includes 39 patients who had histologically negative secondary operations.

salvage surgery, 75 patients (51%) were alive. Subsequent local recurrences were uncommon.

Factors influencing prognosis following salvage surgery included initial clinical stage and axillary nodal status, parameters which not surprisingly were interrelated (table I). 5-year survival after secondary operation was 60% for stage I, 56% for stage II, and 34% for stage III patients. Of 78 patients whose axillae were uninvolved at the time of relapse, 68% survived at least an additional 5 years, whereas the 5-year survival was only 32% for those whose nodes were histologically positive. Patients with T1 or T2 lesions who had recurrences in the breast only had a particularly good prognosis. Patients who had conservative salvage operations did at least as well as those who had radical mastectomies, with 6 of the 10 patients surviving 5 years after being offered a second chance at breast preservation; however, these were carefully selected cases with small, slowly growing recurrences in breasts having few radiosequelae.

In order to quantitate the impact of local failure on the subsequent course of the patients' disease, survival rates were tabulated at 10 years following the date of *primary* therapy for those patients operated for proven local failure compared to those patients not requiring such salvage surgery (table II). It appears that, stage for stage, the 10-year disease-free survival rate is little affected by the development of local recurrence, at least if adequately treated.

Discussion

Despite the availability of convincing long-term survival data demonstrating the equivalent effectiveness of conservative or radical therapy for operable breast cancer [1, 3, 4, 6, 10], concern about the fate of the minority of patients who have recurrences in the preserved breast or axilla following radiation therapy has discouraged many surgeons from endorsing this approach. Although the thrust of our therapeutic efforts should certainly be directed at minimizing local failures, it is nonetheless important that we improve our understanding of the management of such recurrences.

Concerning the morbidity of radical salvage surgery, occasionally performed several years after curative radiation therapy, the complications are understandably somewhat more marked than those we are accustomed to seeing following primary mastectomy. We view this morbidity as acceptable, however, considering that the prolonged wound healing and arm edema seen commonly with the classical radical mastectomy used in this setting can be markedly reduced by the wider application of modified radical mastectomy, simple mastectomy, and conservative salvage operations.

Since the evolution of distant disease will proceed more or less independently of local treatment modalities, a proportion of patients manifesting local-regional failure will prove inoperable due to the recognition of overt metastases. Our high operability rate, especially for early-stage patients, is similar to those reported by other investigations in the literature (table III) [4, 6, 8, 9].

Analysis of survival measured from the time of salvage surgery finds more than half of the patients alive 5 years later, consistent with previously

Table III. Conservative therapy of stage I breast cancer. Operability of local recurrences

Author	Operability	
	n	%
Papillon [9]	21/28	75
Calle et al. [3]	14/17	82
Otmezguine et al. [8]	17/20	85
Delouche and Bachelot [6]	15/22	68
Present series	60/67	90

Table IV. Conservative therapy of stage I breast cancer. Survival after salvage surgery

Author	Number	Survival, %	Follow-up
Papillon [9]	21	67	5 + years
Calle et al. [3]	14	57	4 + years
Delouche and Bachelot [6]	15	67	not stated
Present series	45	60	5 years

published reports from other French centers treating mostly early-stage disease (table IV) [4, 6, 9]. This is in contrast to the prognosis associated with recurrence after radical mastectomy, illustrated by the experience of *Chu* et al. [5]; following radiation treatment of 'isolated' local recurrence after mastectomy, 21% of patients survived for 5 years and only 5% for 10 years. This is confirmed by the study of *Bedwinek* et al. [2], with only 13% of such patients free of disease at 5 years. Clearly, local recurrence after radical surgery is an adverse prognostic indicator, reflecting a more virulent tumor biology and/or a wider disease dissemination than the surgical stage had indicated.

Analysis of 10-year disease-free survival rates following conservative treatment (table II) does not support the notion that recurrence in the intact breast is demonstrably prejudicial to the patients' survival expectancy, provided that the recurrence is operable. Most such recurrences probably do not represent more virulent cancers, but rather a subset of relatively radioresistant tumors, not necessarily a correlate with biologic aggressiveness. Further support for this observation was provided by *Mustakallio* [7], who followed 418 consecutively treated stage I cases, of whom 102 recurred in the irradiated volume. The relative survival curve for the locally recurrent cases was similar to that of the group experiencing no such recurrence, and this equivalence persisted for the entire 25-year duration of the study.

Conclusions

(1) Following conservative treatment, about 80 % of local failures are operable.

(2) Morbidity of salvage surgery, though significant, is acceptable.

(3) Treated local failure has little demonstrable effect on 10-year survival rates.

(4) More than 50 % of patients survive at least 5 years following salvage surgery.

(5) Survival after salvage surgery depends upon the *original* clinical stage and the presence or absence of involved nodes in the operative specimen.

(6) The prognosis of patients with local recurrences after conservative treatment is much better than the outlook following local recurrence after radical surgery; it is thus inappropriate to compare recurrence rates after the two disparate forms of treatment.

References

1   Amalric R.; Santamaria, F.; Robert, F. et al.: Radiation therapy with or without primary limited surgery for operable breast cancer: a 20-year experience at the Marseilles Cancer Institute. Cancer *49:* 30 (1982).

2   Bedwinek, M.M.; Lee, J.; Fineberg, B.; Ocwieza, M.: Prognostic indicators in patients with isolated local-regional recurrences of breast cancer. Cancer *47:* 2232 (1981).

3   Calle, R.; Pilleron, J.P.; Schlienger, P.; Vilcoq, J.R.: Conservative management of operable breast cancer. Ten years' experience at the Fondation Curie. Cancer *42:* 2045 (1978).

4   Calle, R.; Pilleron, J.P.: Radiation therapy, with and without lumpectomy, for operable breast cancer. Breast *5/4:* 2 (1979).

5   Chu, F.C.H.; Lin, F.; Kim, J.H.; Huh, S.H.; Gormatis, C.J.: Locally recurrent carcinoma of the breast: results of radiation therapy. Cancer *37:* 2677 (1976).

6   Delouche, G.; Bachelot, F.: Tumorectomie et radiothérapie pour les petits cancers du sein opérables d'emblée. Résultats à 5 et 10 ans. J. eur. Radiothér. *1:* 133 (1980).

7   Mustakallio, S.; Conservative treatment of breast carcinoma. Review of 25-year follow-up. Clin. Radiol. *23:* 110 (1972).

8   Otmezguine, Y. et al.: Etude des récidives parmi 202 cancéreuses du sein traitées conservativement par radiothérapie. J. eur. Radiothér. *1:* 115 (1980).

9   Papillon, J.: Conservative treatments of early breast cancer by tumorectomy and irradiation; in Castro, Current concepts in breast cancer and tumor immunology, p. 117 (Huber, Berne 1974).

10   Pierquin, B.; Owen, R.; Maylin, C. et al.: Radical radiaton therapy of breast cancer. Int. J. Radiat. Oncol. Biol. Phys. *6:* 17 (1980).

J. M. Kurtz, MD, Swedish Hospital Tumor Institute, Seattle, WA 98104 (USA)

Front. Radiat. Ther. Onc., vol. 17, pp. 91–101 (Karger, Basel 1983)

Conservative Surgery and Radiation Therapy in the Treatment of Operable Breast Cancer

Roy M. Clark

Princess Margaret Hospital, Toronto, Ont., Canada

Introduction

Seldom in the history of medicine have we witnessed so much dedication to the preservation of the status quo in the surgical treatment of breast cancer. The defence of the radical mastectomy has continued unabated since 1894 when *Halstead* [4] first published his results. His interpretation of cure was grossly inadequate and the results indicated a reduction in local recurrence without a notable increase in survival. Even today many surgeons still defer to a procedure which at least includes total mastectomy. Radiation oncologists have also been somewhat reluctant to abdicate their support of routine postoperative irradiation to the breast area and regional nodes. They consistently disregard numerous reports indicating that although the incidence of local recurrence is reduced, there is again, no significant effect on survival.

Over the years, many radiation oncologists and a few intrepid surgeons have become convinced that the ultimate results of a variety of techniques, ranging from radical mastectomy to simple local tumor excision, differ very little. Studies of conservative treatment are usually retrospective. In 1982, when sophisticated statistical analysis reigns supreme, the mere mention of a retrospective study smacks of impiety. The prospective randomized study is having its day, but its objectives need close inspection. It has been said by *Gehan and Freireich* [3] that all knowledge is historical and modifications to the body of knowledge are made as new evidence accumulates. The prospective randomized study compares treatments which are considered to be equivalent. The design of this type of study is therefore often based on knowledge derived from nonrandomized retrospective studies. Present studies incorporating conservative management could never have been accepted ethically, if a few pioneers had not already produced retrospective reports on patients they had treated in this manner.

A comparison of equivalent treatments will refine treatment, but will not be responsible for major advances. It is the sudden leap forward that is really required in the treatment of this disease. This will not come from the prospective randomized approach.

There is sufficient information derived from this study to demonstrate that a more positive movement towards conservative management is indicated and should provide the basis for future advances.

Patients and Methods

This study includes 680 patients treated by partial mastectomy and referred to the Princess Margaret Hospital between January 1958 and December 1978. 'Partial mastectomy' includes wedge resection, excisional biopsy, segmental resection and lumpectomy. None of these patients had clinical evidence of nodal involvement in the axilla or supraclavicular regions. The majority did not have an axillary dissection, but those that did were still included whether the nodes were positive or not. It has been established that clinically, the false-negative rate for metastatic disease in axillary nodes may be as high as 40 % [1]. These patients, therefore, represent a mixture of pathological stage I and II disease. Patients over 75 years of age were excluded as they were unlikely to provide data for extended follow-up; otherwise the distribution was typical with 23 % aged 65–75 at diagnosis and 24 % under 45. In recent years there has been a marked increase in the number of patients treated conservatively at this hospital, rising from 235 patients treated the first 16 years of this study, to 445 treated during the last 5 years. Indeed, at the present time, we have now accumulated almost 1,000 patients who have been treated in this manner.

The trend towards conservative treatment became more marked from 1973 onwards, and at the same time, the use of postoperative radiation therapy became less standard and the technique more variable. In the earlier period most of the patients, following partial mastectomy, received postoperative irradiation to the breast and regional nodes but more recently, 154 patients were treated by excision only with no irradiation and 195 received radiation therapy to the breast only. No other adjuvant therapy was given.

If relapse occurred, subsequent treatment was sequential depending on the site of relapse. If possible, the policy of breast conservation was continued. If relapse occurred in axillary nodes and the breast remained clinically free of disease, only an axillary dissection was performed. Relapse in the breast with no evidence of disease in regional nodes was again treated by partial mastectomy if feasible. Of necessity, some patients proceeded to simple or modified radical mastectomies because of the breast size or extent of relapse in the breast or axilla.

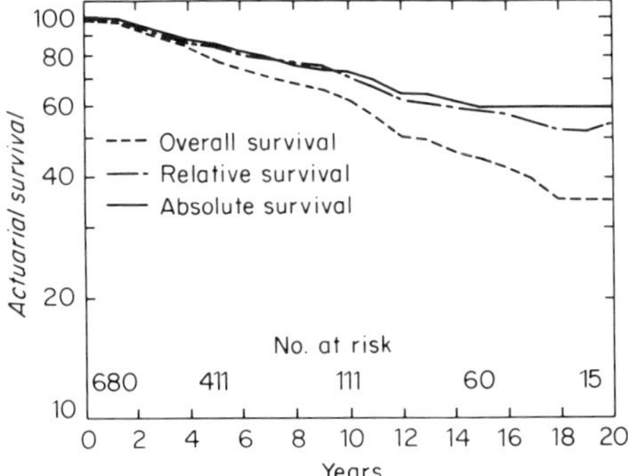

Yrs. after diagnosis	Overall survival	Relative survival	Absolute survival
5	78%	83%	83%
10	62%	71%	73%
15	44%	57%	59%
20	35%	53%	59%

Fig. 1. Overall actuarial survival.

Radiation Technique

To preserve a good cosmetic and symptomatic result, radiation skin reactions were avoided and the dose of radiation was optimized to prevent significant fibrosis in the beast. All but 20 patients received a dose of 4,000 rad given by ^{60}Co over a period of 3 weeks in 16 daily treatments In 43% of the patients, a boost of 500 rad was given to the primary site split into two consecutive daily doses given during the treatment to the other fields, using a direct field with either ^{60}Co, or 250 kV orthovoltage therapy. The breast was treated by a pair of parallel opposed fields, tangential to the chest wall, with no bolus. The curvature was compensated by wedges.

Statistical Methods

In this series, relapse implies first relapse at the site specified with no evidence of disease elsewhere at that time. Local relapse is defined as disease presenting within a tissue volume which includes the breast and all ipsilateral regional node areas. Patients with local and distant relapse simultaneously are recorded as distant relapse. Absolute survival rates were obtained by censoring those patients whose deaths were due to causes other than breast cancer.

Table I. Pathological T and N staging

	Patients, n	%
T (pathological)		
T_{1S}	4	1
T_1	312	46
T_2	144	21
T_3	7 ⎫	⎫
T_4	3 ⎪	⎪
Multifocal	22 ⎬ 37	5 ⎬ 32
Bilateral (at diagnosis)	5 ⎪	⎪
Tx	183 ⎭	27 ⎭
Total	680	100
N (pathological)		
N_0	48	7 ⎫ 11
N_1	29	4 ⎭
No axillary dissection	603	89
Total	680	100

Results

The overall actuarial survival at 5 years was 78% and at 10 years 62% (fig. 1). Relative survivals were 83 and 71%, respectively. The absolute survival was similar to the relative indicating the absence of serious iatrogenic disease. 8 patients died of other malignancies including 2 that may have been related to radiation therapy, although this is only a remote possibility. 1 had acute granulocytic leukaemia and the other an adenocarcinoma of the right lung apex, which was within the irradiated volume. 5 patients had bilateral disease at diagnosis and of the rest, 15 or 2.2% have now developed a second primary in the opposite breast. This figure is not in excess of that commonly quoted in the literature [5].

An accurate statement of clinical tumor size was not possible in approximately 50% of patients due to incomplete information. Pathological T staging was more accurate with 27% assigned to (Tx) (table I). The

Table II. Pathological T staging for no radiation group

T (pathological)	Patients, n	%
T_{is}	3	2
T_1	87	57
T_2	22	14
T_3	1	
T_4	1	
Multifocal	4	8 → 5
Bilateral	2	
Tx	34	22
Total	154	100

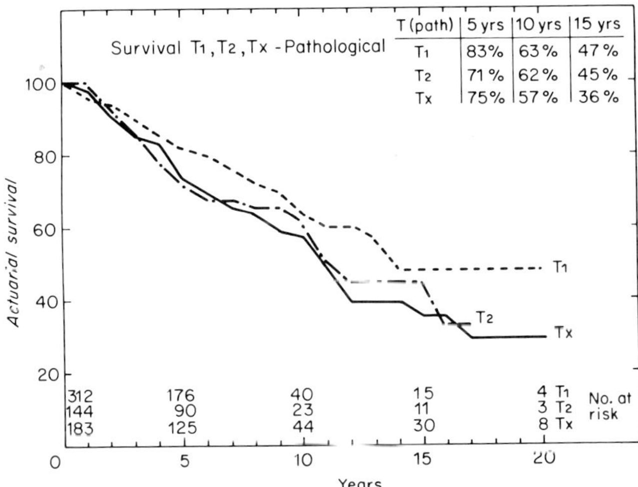

Fig. 2. Survival by pathological T stage.

necessity for accurate assessment rather than a deferred estimate cannot be overemphasized if it is intended to use staging in the selection of treatment groups.

Reviewing the pathological staging, 21% had T2 tumors and another 5% either T3, T4, multifocal or bilateral disease. The nodal status could not be given in 89% of patients, because no axillary dissection was performed (table I).

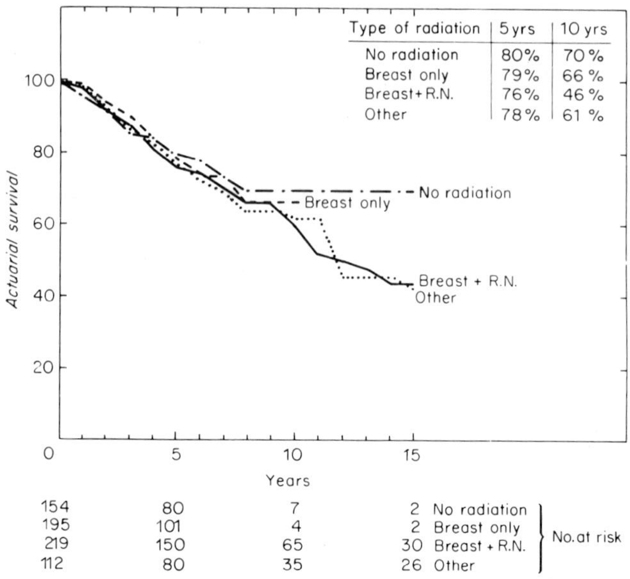

Fig. 3. Survival by type of radiation (no statistical significance between groups).

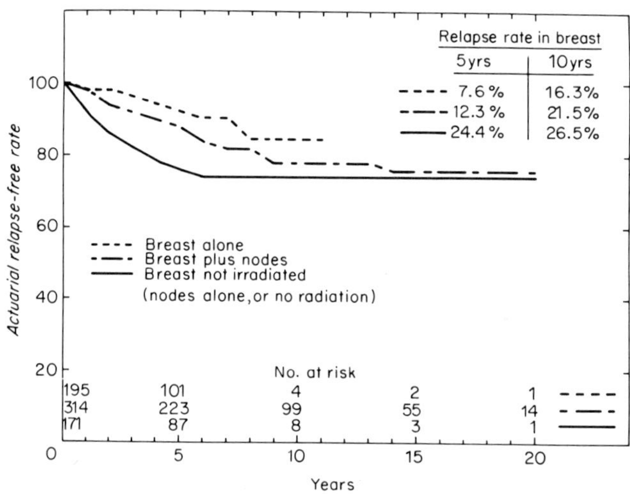

Fig. 4. Relapse rate in breast by radiation method. Breast alone versus breast plus nodes; p = 0.068. Breast not irradiated versus breast alone or breast plus nodes; p = <0.0005.

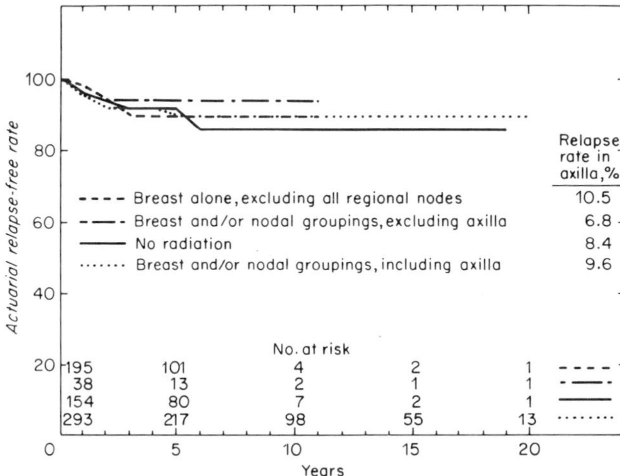

Fig. 5. Relapse rate in axilla by method of treatment.

It should also be noted that even amongst the 154 patients who had no radiation 14% were T2, indicating that this method of treatment was not specifically selected for patients with only minimal disease (table II).

When comparing survival with tumor size, there was no significant difference in survival by T stage, but patients with pathological T1 tumors had an actuarial survival rate of 83% at 5 years and 63% at 10 years (fig. 2).

There was no difference in survival by volume irradiated or if no radiation was given. This point needs emphasizing, in that we are saying that patients who have been treated by a partial mastectomy only, with no other treatment, have the same survival at 10 years as those who were irradiated (fig. 3).

Conservative treatment is basically aimed at preserving the breast. Therefore, it is of fundamental importance to consider relapse in the breast. In those patients where the breast only was irradiated, the relapse rate was 7.6% at 5 years. If the breast and any nodal grouping was irradiated the relapse rate was 12.3%. With no radiation to the breast, the relapse rate was 24.4%, in spite of the fact that in this group there was a larger proportion of patients with more favourable disease. By 10 years the relapse rates rose to 16.3, 21.5 and 26.5%, respectively. Subsequently, a plateau was reached in all groups (fig. 4).

Recurrence in any other part of the breast remote from the original primary site was exceptional and occurred in only 3 instances. Multicentric

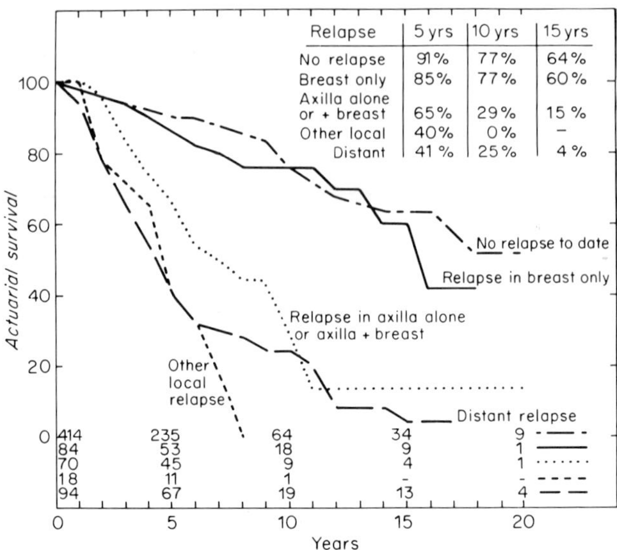

Fig. 6. Comparison of survival from diagnosis for patients with no relapse, in breast only, relapse in axilla alone or with breast, other local relapse, and with distant relapse. No relapse versus breast relapse; p = 0.368. Breast relapse versus axillary relapse; p = 0.002.

disease has therefore not influenced our pattern of recurrence significantly. The effect of a radiation boost to the primary site was to reduce the relapse rate at 5 years, but at 10 years there was no difference.

The axillary relapse rate was approximately 10% at 5 years and reached a plateau subsequently whether radiation was given to the breast alone, axilla in addition or when no radiation was given at all. If we accept the clinical false-negative rate of 40% for axillary involvement, this figure is much lower than expected for those receiving no treatment to the axilla (fig. 5).

One of the most interesting aspects of this study was the effect of relapse on survival. Patients who relapse only in the breast have the same survival as patients who have never relapsed at any site. Relapse in the breast alone is therefore not detrimental to survival (fig. 6).

At the date of analysis, the estimate of the overall relapse-free rate for the entire group suggests a cured population if we look at the flat tail of the curve, but this cannot be inferred from the relative and absolute survival curves previously shown (fig. 7).

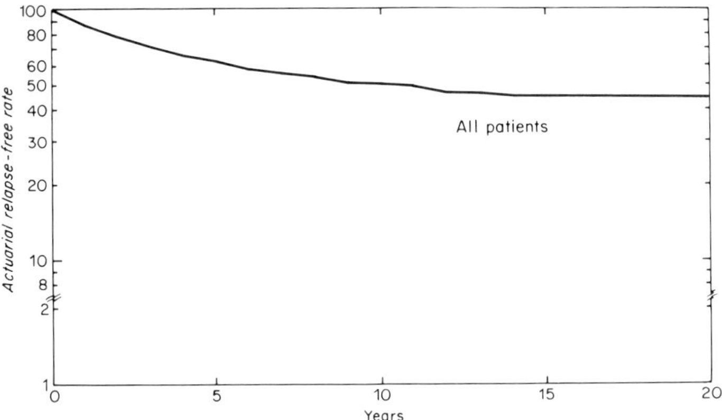

Fig. 7. Overall relapse-free rate.

Discussion

The ultimate parameter of successful treatment is survival. In this series, the relative survival of 71% at 10 years compared favourably with reported survival rates for radical surgery. It has also been demonstrated that postoperatve irradiation does not influence survival or axillary relapse. It does, however, significantly decrease relapse within the breast if one examines the treatment groups with the log rank test.

The majority of patients in this series did not have wide excisions and as we had no control over the primary surgery, it was impossible to assess the completeness of excision retrospectively. Unfortunately, if relapse does occur in the breast a total mastectomy may be required to achieve control, although a further local excision may be possible if the relapse is small compared with the size of the breast. If the initial concept is to preserve the breast, providing this is not detrimental to survival, relapse in the breast must be avoided because in this series 76% of those relapsing in the breast required some form of total mastectomy.

Excessively radical radiation therapy may, in the long term, be as destructive as the radical surgery it is intended to replace. Severe skin reactions must be avoided, or unsightly telangiectasia will appear in later years, producing a poor cosmetic result. A heavily irradiated breast with the resultant fibrosis may also produce extreme discomfort.

As only 3 patients relapsed outside the original primary site within the breast, we do not feel that a higher dose of radiation to the entire breast is required. The present boosting dose delayed relapse, but at 10 years the rate was the same as in the no radiation group. As the relapse rate was similar for T1 and T2 tumors, there is no indication that smaller tumors need not receive a boost. The dose to this site will therefore be increased either by external radiation or an interstitial implant.

An axillary relapse rate of 10% in a subgroup, where no surgical or radiation treatment was given, is significantly low when compared with the accepted false-negative rate of 40% for the clinical assessment of axillary nodal involvement. Irradiation of the regional nodes will therefore not be continued. This will also eliminate the necessity for careful field matching to avoid high dose areas in the breast, which inevitably lead to subcutaneous fibrosis and late skin changes. As part of the routine treatment, axillary dissections are now being performed in addition to partial mastectomy. This is basically to select patients who require adjuvant therapy because we acknowledge that axillary dissection has prognostic but no therapeutic value.

Internal mammary lymphoscintigraphy is used routinely in the work-up of our patients and we have previously demonstrated that patients in this study with positive internal mammary lymphoscintigrams had a significantly reduced survival [2]. These patients will now receive adjuvant therapy. At the present time, we have also added axillary lymphoscintigraphy, which is performed prior to any surgery. We hope that this will be sufficiently accurate in the detection of nodal metastases to render even an axillary dissection unnecessary for patients with clinically negative axillae.

Finally, I would like to return to the question of prospective randomized studies. In Ontario, because we require fully informed consent, it has become increasingly difficult to recruit patients for this type of study. To detect a significant statistical difference between treatment arms for a group of patients with a relatively good survival, large numbers and a long follow-up period are also essential. This compounds the problem.

Pre-randomization has been presented as an alternative to discussing the merits of the treatments under consideration with the patient. I am not sure that this is ethically acceptable and also doubt, in an era of increasing patient awareness of all aspects of medical treatment, that one can really expect a discerning patient to approve our lack of decision when we are asked for a frank expression of our views on what is considered to be the best method of treatment. The physician is expected to be an arbiter and may not be allowed to relegate this role to a study. Patient-doctor relationships are traditionally sacrosanct and may be negated by randomized studies.

References

1 Cancer Research Campaign Working Party: Cancer research campaign (King's/Cambridge) trial for early breast cancer. Lancet *ii:* 55–60 (1980).
2 Ege, G.N.; Clark, R.M.: Internal mammary lymphoscintigraphy in the conservative surgical management of breast carcinoma. Clin. Radiol. *31:* 559–563 (1980).
3 Gehan, E.A.; Freireich, E.J.: Cancer clinical trials. A rational basis for use of historical controls. Semin. Oncol. *8:* 430–436 (1981).
4 Halstead, W.S.: The results of operations for the cure of cancer of the breast performed at the Johns Hopkins Hospital from June 1889 to January 1894. Johns Hopkins Hosp. Rep. *4:* 297–350 (1894-5).
5 Leis, P.H.: Managing the remaining breast. Cancer *46:* 1026–1030 (1980).

R.M.Clark, MD, Senior Radiation Oncologist, Princess Margaret Hospital, Toronto, Ont. M4X 1K9 (Canada)

Front. Radiat. Ther. Onc., vol. 17, pp. 102–109 (Karger, Basel 1983)

Conservation Surgery and Radiotherapy in the Treatment of Localized Breast Cancer

A Retrospective Analysis

Nemetallah A. Ghossein[a], *Jacques R. Vilcoq*[b], *Patricia Stacey*[a], *Robert Calle*[b,1]

[a] Department of Radiotherapy, Albert Einstein College of Medicine, Yeshiva University, Bronx, N.Y., USA, and [b] Institute Curie, Paris, France

Introduction

There is an ongoing controversy regarding the most appropriate treatment for localized breast cancer. Over the years, there has been a steady trend toward less radical procedures. For the past three to four decades, we have witnessed a shifting from the supraradical to radical mastectomy and from radical mastectomy to modified radical mastectomy. Now there is a definite shift towards breast-preserving procedures in the form of quadrantectomy and tumorectomy. At each stage controversies arose because the results of these different methods appear to be similar.

Tumorectomy, which essentially means gross removal of the tumor mass with a small margin of surrounding normal breast tissue, is the least deforming of these treatment modalities.

The present work is a cooperative study between the Institute Curie (IC) in Paris, France and the Albert Einstein College of Medicine (AECOM) in New York City.

Although tumorectomy followed by radiotherapy has been a well-established procedure for the treatment of localized breast cancer in Europe [3, 8] and Canada [9] for many years, few surgeons in the United States offered this modality to their patients as an alternative to mastectomy.

[1] The authors would like to thank *Grace Baione* for her secretarial help in the preparation of this manuscript.

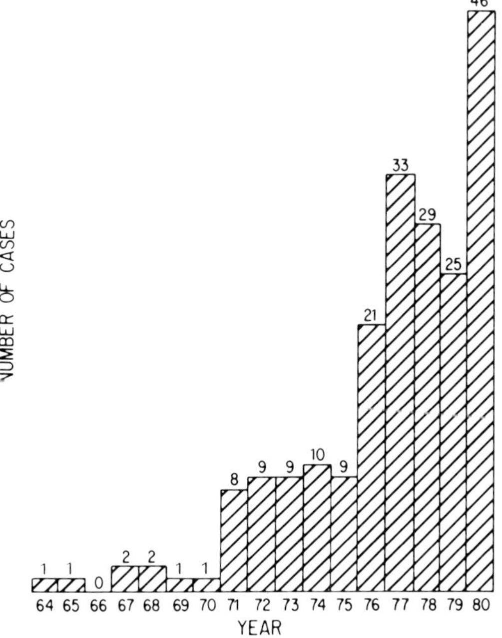

Fig. 1. Tumorectomy and radiotherapy for surgically operable breast cancer number of patients by year.

At AECOM, like most centers in the United States, a few patients were referred for this breast-preserving procedure. In the early 1970s more patients became aware of this alternative through the news media and the number of patients seeking this form of treatment increased sharply (fig. 1).

Material and Method

There was a total of 307 patients with a minimum follow-up of 5 years: 233 from IC and 74 from AECOM. 136 patients had a minimum follow-up of 10 years. All patients had tumorectomy followed by radiotherapy using a mega-voltage unit (usually a Cobalt 60 unit) and were staged according to the TNM classification of the International Union Against Cancer (UICC) [10]. The patients characteristics are shown in table I. The average age of patients from IC is only 46 years, whereas that of the AECOM group is 60. This is due to the fact that many of the AECOM patients were treated by this conservative method because they were considered to be medically inoperable due to age associated illnesses. The treatment protocol was described previously [2, 5]. In order to avoid significant deformity of the breast,

Table I. Tumorectomy and radiotherapy: characteristics of patients studied

	Stage	Maximum age	Average age	Minimum follow-up period, years	
		years	years	5	10
IC	T_1–T_2 (≤ 3 cm) N_0, N_1a	70	46	233	120
AECOM	T_1–T_2 small T_3 (≤ 6 cm) N_0–N_1a, N_1b	any age	60	74	16
Total				307	136

tumorectomy at IC was performed only on those patients with tumor ≤ 3 cm. (T_1 and small T_2 tumors) and with clinically negative axilla (N_0). At AECOM, the indication for tumorectomy was more liberal. It was done on patients who had larger tumors (≤ 6 cm) and with or without palpable but mobile axillary nodes (T_1–T_2 and small T_3, N_0– N_1b).

Following tumorectomy a tumor dose of 5,000–5,500 rad was usually given to the entire breast in 5–6 weeks. An additional 1,000–2,000 rad was given to the area of tumorectomy through reduced portals, mostly through decubitus fields. The supra- and infraclavicular regions received about 5,000 rad given dose and the axilla 5,000-rad tumor dose. Patients with clinically suspicious axillary nodes received an additional 1,000–2,000 rad to the lower axilla.

Loco-regional failure is defined as recurrence in the breast and/or homolateral axilla or supraclavicular lymph nodes.

Results

The absolute survival free of disease (NED) at 5 years for patients with T_1 stage is 91%. The survival from the two centers is similar (92 and 86%, respectively). Of those who were alive free of disease, 96% had a preserved breast.

The survival for the patients with T_2 stage is 76%. It is significantly better for the IC patients because the AECOM group had patients with more advanced tumors and, furthermore, about 10% of them died of intercurrent diseases but were considered to have died of cancer. These results are shown in table II.

In table III is shown the incidence of the first clinical relapse after the initial treatment as well as death from intercurrent diseases at the last

Table II. Breast carcinoma, tumorectomy and radiotherapy: results of treatment from Institute Curie (IC), Paris, and Albert Einstein College of Medicine (AECOM), New York

	Stage	Number of patients	Absolute survival NED	Alive NED with preserved breast
IC	$T_1 N_0$	150	138/150 (92%)	133/138 (96%)
AECOM	$T_1 N_0-N_1 b$	29	25/29 (86%)	24/25 (96%)
Total		179	163/179 (91%)	157/163 (96%)
IC	$T_2 N_0$ (≤ 3 cm)	83	69/83 (83%)	63/69 (91%)
AECOM	T_2-T_3 (≤ 6 cm) $N_0-N_1 b$	45	28/45 (62%)	27/28 (96%)
Total		128	97/128 (76%)	90/97 (93%)

Minimal follow-up: 5 years.

Table III. Breast carcinoma, tumorectomy and radiotherapy: first clinical relapse after initial treatment

	IC (n = 233)	AECOM (n = 74)
Loco-regional	20 (8%)	5 (7%)
Distant metastases	15 (6%)	10 (13%)
Second primary	1 (0.5%)	7[a] (9%)
Intercurrent disease	1 (0.5%)	7 (9%)
Lost to follow-up	1 (0.5%)	1 (1%)

Minimum follow-up: 5 years.
[a] 4 outside breast, 3 in opposite breast.

follow-up. Loco-regional failure is similar in the two groups and is about 8% at 5 years.

The result of treatment at 10 years is shown in table IV. The absolute survival NED is 77% for IC patients. But it is only 31% for the AECOM group. This is due to the fact that the majority of patients treated in the early period at AECOM were unfit for surgical resection because of medical illnesses and therefore, deaths from intercurrent diseases was high (50%)

Table IV. Tumorectomy and radiotherapy: results of treatment from Institute Curie (IC), Paris, and Albert Einstein College of Medicine (AECOM), New York, minimum follow-up 10 years

	Stage	Number of patients	Absolute survival NED	Alive (NED) with breast preserved	Dead or alive with cancer	Dead of intercurrent disease
IC	T_1-T_2 ($\leq$ 3 cm) N_0	120	92/120 (77%)	82/92 (89%)	21/120 (18%)	7/120 (6%)
AECOM	$T_1-T_2-T_3$ ($\leq$ 6 cm) N_0-N_1b	16	5/16 (31%)	4/5	3/16 (19%)	8/16 (50%)

Table V. Breast carcinoma, tumorectomy and radiotherapy: survival after first loco-regional recurrrence in patients with a minimum follow-up of 10 years (Institute Curie)

	Number of patients	Alive NED
Before 5 years	14	8
After 5 years	7	5
Total	21/120 (17%)	13/21 (62%)

The long-term survival of patients who developed loco-regional failure was determined in the IC group only, because this group did not have a significant number of patients who died of intercurrent illnesses. The data are shown in table V. Almost two thirds of those who developed loco-regional recurrences were alive with a minimum follow-up of 10 years. The presence of histologically proven recurrences in the axilla appears to have an ominous prognosis. Over 85% of those patients, who had recurrences in the breast only, were alive at 5 years, whereas less than half of those who had positive axillary nodes at the time of salvage surgery were alive.

The cosmetic results at 5 years for the two series were similar and were excellent or good in 98% of the patients. Significant radiation sequelae were negligible.

Table VI. Tumorectomy and radiotherapy: incidence of local recurrence according to the microscopic involvement of the margin of resection

Stage	Number of cases	Margin positive	Local recurrence	Margin negative	Local recurrence
T_1	29	10/29 (35%)	1/10 (10%)	19/29 (65%)	1/19 (5%)
T_2	37	17/37 (46%)	3/17 (18%)	20/37 (54%)	1/20 (5%)
T_3 (≤ 6 cm)	8	5/8 (–)	0/5 (–)	3/8 (–)	1/3 (–)
Total	74	32/74 (43%)	4/32 (12%)	42/74 (57%)	3/42 (7%)

Minimum follow-up: 5 years.

Discussion

There now is an extensive body of evidence [1, 3, 6, 7, 12] to show that tumorectomy followed by adequate doses of radiotherapy is not only an alternative to mastectomy but is the treatment modality of choice for patients with localized breast cancer if the tumorectomy can be done without distortion of the breast and radiotherapy can be given without great technical difficulties. An important question which should be answered is the nature of the conservative procedure to be performed. Is it necessary to do a wide breast resection, which is the case with quadrantectomy, with its associated deformity particularly in lesions of the inner quadrants of the breasts, or is it sufficient to perform removal of the tumor with 1 or 2 cm of surrounding grossly normal breast tissue? In a recent randomized study [11] between radical mastectomy and quadrantectomy and axillary dissection followed by postoperative radiotherapy to the breast for patients with T_1N_0 tumor, there was no advantage in favor of the radical mastectomy group, either in disease-free or overall survival. Of interest is that the absolute disease-free survival at 5 years, reported in our present study for patients with T_1N_0 lesions, is almost identical to the actuarial survival at 7 years reported for patients who were treated by quadrantectomy and axillary dissection. This appears to indicate that adequate dose radiotherapy to the breast following gross tumor removal may be quite sufficient to irradicate microscopic disease obviating the need for quadrantectomy. We have analyzed the incidence of local recurrence according to the microscopic involvement of the surgical margin by cancer at the time of tumorectomy. This study was performed on the 74 patients of AECOM. 43% had positive margin and 57% had negative margin on histological examination. Although the local recurrence rate was somewhat higher for those patients with a positive margin (12% compared to 7%), this difference is not statistically significant (table VI). It is an indication that adequate postoperative irradiation to the breast can sterilize the incompletely resected tumor [5].

Lastly, although it is known that local recurrence following mastectomy is associated with poor prognosis [4], this does not appear to be the case when patients are treated by tumorectomy [12]. Salvage surgery appears to be extremely effective since about two thirds of our patients who developed loco-regional recurrence were alive at 10 years.

In conclusion, this study indicates that mastectomy is an unnecessary mutilitation which should be avoided, if at all possible, for patients with localized breast cancer which could be removed by tumorectomy and in whom postoperative radiotherapy can be delivered without great technical difficulties.

References

1   Alpert, S.; Ghossein, N.A.; Stacey, P.; Migliorelli, F.A.; Efron, G.; Krishnaswamy, V.: Primary management of operable breast cancer by minimal surgery and radiotherapy. Cancer *42:* 2054–2058 (1978).
2   Calle, R.; Fletcher, G.H.; Peirquin, B.: Les bases de la radiothérapie, curative des épithéliomas mammaires. J. Radiol. Electrol. Méd. nucl. *54:* 929–938 (1973).
3   Calle, R.; Pilleron, J.P.; Schlienger, P.; Vilcoq, J.R.: Conservative management of operable breast cancer. Ten years experience at the Foundation Curie. Cancer *42:* 2045–2053 (1978).
4   Donegan, W.L.; Perez-Mesa, C.M.; Watson, F.R.: A biostatistical study of locally recurrent breast carcinoma. Surgery Gynec. Obstet. *122:* 529–540 (1966).
5   Ghossein, N.A.; Stacey, P.; Alpert, S.; Ager, P.H.; Krishnaswamy, V.: Local control of breast cancer with tumorectomy plus radiotherapy or radiotherapy alone. Radiology *121:* 455–459 (1976).
6   Harris, J.R.; Levene, M.B.; Hellman, S.: The role of radiation therapy in the primary treatment of carcinoma of the breast. Semin. Oncol. *5:* 403–416 (1978).

7   Montague, E.D.; Gutierrez, A.E.; Barker, J.L.; Tapley, N.D.; Fletcher, G.H.: Conservation surgery and irradiation for the treatment of favorable breast cancer. Cancer *43:* 1058–1061 (1979).
8   Mustakalio, S.: Conservative treatment of breast carcinoma. Clin. Radiol. *23:* 110–116 (1972).
9   Peters, V.: Wedge resection with or without radiation in early breast cancer. Int. J. Radiat. Oncol. Biol. Phys. *2:* 1151–1156 (1977).
10   Union Internationale Contre le Cancer: TNM Classification of malignant tumors (UICC, Geneva 1974).
11   Veronesi, U.; Saccozzi, R.; Del Vecchio, M.; Banfi, A.L.; Clemente, C. et al.: Comparing radical mastectomy with quadrantectomy, axillary dissection and radiotherapy in patients with small cancers of the breast. New Engl. J. Med. *305:* 6–11 (1981).
12   Vilcoq, J.R.; Calle, R.; Stacey, P.; Ghossein, N.A.: The outcome of treatment by tumorectomy and radiotherapy of patients with operable breast cancer. Int. J. Radiat. Oncol. Biol. Phys. *7:* 1327–1332 (1981).

N.A. Ghossein, MD, 1180 Morris Park Avenue, Bronx, NY 10461 (USA)

Front. Radiat. Ther. Onc., vol. 17, pp. 110–114 (Karger, Basel 1983)

Discussion

Moderator Cantril: I note that there is a considerable variation in treatment technique. It ranges from boost to no boost, but not so much the dose. There seems to be a good deal of disagreement as to whether the lymph nodes need to be treated, and certainly discussing this matter with my colleagues here in San Francisco, that seems to be a matter of dispute. Our first speaker told us that the pendulous breasts were a reason not to do this procedure, and I think all of the other 4 disagreed with him. There still remain some unresolved questions.

Montague (Houston): With regards to the size of the breast, I do think that there are some women whose breasts are so big that unless you have some technical equipment like boxes and things in which to put them, it becomes very difficult to treat. When we have that type of breast size, we do tell them to have a mastectomy. We recently had a woman whose breasts were so big that in our treatment position we would be treating the upper outer quadrant of the abdomen. There is no point, I think, to that because we are really only doing this for cosmetic effect. When it is technically too difficult, we should tell the patient that she is better suited for a mastectomy. When breasts are that big, most patients are really quite happy not only to have a mastectomy on that side but sometimes have something done about the other side, as Dr. *Westdahl* described today. With reference to the axilla or regional nodes, I agree with *Clark* that there are a great many things about axillary nodes and regional lymphatics that we don't yet know, but it is true that there is some derangement of facts with reference to axillary recurrence. He described that 10 % of the patients who had no treatment to the axilla recurred in the axilla, whereas you would expect 40 % at least to recur in the axilla because that's the amount of error in clinical estimation of the axilla. It is interesting that this experience at the Princess Margaret is corroborated by the NSADT study. That's where the 40 % error in estimated axillary recurrence was established. In the radical mastectomy group 40 % had pathologically positive nodes whereas they were all clinically negative. You would think that the incidence of recurrent disease in the axilla in the total mastectomy group alone would be something like 30 or 40 %, but it wasn't. At the end of 9 years, it was still 15 or 16 %. We have 9 years of follow-up and only 15 % of the patients without treatment to the axilla by any means have developed no growth in the axilla. Obviously there is a great deal biologically that we don't understand about patients with breast cancer. The difference between the 15 % and the 40 % must be taking care of their own axillary nodes in some way.

Ghossein (New York): I think a good number of patients with metastasis in the axilla – although clinically N-O, histologically are more than 3 nodes – would develop distant metastasis and are counted as dead of distant disease and local recurrence. This is very crucial. Perhaps we are shifting them from a group where we do not observe local recurrence in the axilla because they have been grouped already in the group with disseminated disease rather than local recurrence. They have to live long enough without disseminated disease to be included into the recurrence in the axilla proper. I think this is perhaps a little bit biased; that's why the two numbers don't add together.

Montague: I would add one more comment to that. If you expect an incidence of axillary failure with 10 %, and if you can avoid it, could one take the option of trying to cure their patient? For me I think the 10 % recurrence in the axilla by leaving it untreated is too much, so I personally would not leave the axilla untreated. I might if the recurrence rate in the axilla was 1 % or 2 %, but 10 % would be too much failure because a radical mastectomy done for operable axillary disease doesn't have a 10 % failure rate in the axilla; it's about 1.5 %. If we don't do as good a job as surgery, then our surgeons are going to say, 'Well, there's no reason to do conservative surgery if we get better results with radical mastectomy'. So I don't agree in part, then, with the conclusion that Dr. *Clark* made, because I wouldn't leave the axilla untreated.

Cantril (San Francisco): Untreated by what – either surgery or radiotherapy?

Montague: Yes, as I said, you have to decide what you are going to do. We're doing it with surgery, but you can certainly do it just as successfully with radiation therapy as long as the disease is clinically negative.

Dymott (San Francisco): I just want to comment that I find this interesting in that there is a discrepancy between what we know about the clinically false negative axilla and what the course seems to be. We already know in the case with the internal mammary nodes, the surgically positive rate is much higher than we actually see in the rate of internal mammary node recurrence in mastectomy patients who have not been irradiated. *Fisher* wrote about the number of nodes removed from the axilla, during the radical mastectomy and correlated this with the 1.4 % axillary recurrences. The paper intimates that if one gets up to 10 negative nodes from the axilla by actually sampling, then essentially there are no axillary recurrences. Actually their recurrence number was lower than with the radical mastectomy.

Montague: There is something in the way that *Fisher* presents those data. If you look at the total mastectomy recurrence in the axilla, it is true it was 0.8 %, I think, in the last, which is lower. But the number of patients who have axillary growth are not included in that 0.8 %, because as part of the study Dr. *Fisher* says that if you don't treat the axilla and if the axillary recurrence develops, you then treat it with an axillary dissection. 0.8 % of the patients failed in the axilla after axillary dissection. But they did not include the 16 % of patients who had axillary growth. For us that would have been an axillary recurrence had we treated the axilla. They did not treat the axilla. You have to look at that very carefully because that axillary regrowth (axillary recurrence rate) did not include the 16 % of patients who had axillary regrowth.

Demare (Honolulu): We have heard the words, 'excisional biopsy', 'wedge resection', 'quadrantectomy', 'tylectomy', 'wide local excision', 'tumorectomy', 'segmental resection', 'partial mastectomy'. Is there an optimal surgical procedure before irradiation and what is it?

Clark (Toronto): All the patients in Toronto are now receiving a very minimal surgical excision with a very, very small margin of normal tissue, so there are no longer quadrantectomies, segmentectomies, that type of thing being done. In fact often it is rather embarrassing to meet 2 patients in your waiting room, one of whom has had a modified radical and the other has had just a lumpectomy. She has seen her partner's scar and compared it with her own which may only be 2 or 3 cm long, and she wants to know why there is such a discrepancy in treatment in 1982. I think the only thing you can say is that some people still believe in modified radical mastectomies, but we don't.

Cantril: Would the whole panel agree with that, basically as little surgery as possible?

Ghossein: I analyzed about 50 patients referred to us with operations described as tylectomy, wide resection, local resection. In reality what happens is the surgeon takes about 1 cm margin about the gross nodule; only the semantics vary. A quadrantectomy, however, can be quite a large procedure.

Sherman (San Francisco): All the panelists' presentations were a series of patients who did or did not have axillary nodes but basically did not receive chemotherapy. It's a different situation if patients do get chemotherapy. Whether we do believe the data or not, the drugs go in. I wonder if each of the panelists would give their philosophy about treating the regional lymphatics in a woman who is going to retain her breast but has had surgical proof that there is axillary node involvement and is going to receive chemotherapy, whether CMF or an adriamycin-containing regimen. Do you treat the nodes? And if you do, which nodes do you treat?

Clark: If the axillary nodes are positive, we treat the internal mammary and the supraclavicular nodes.

Ghossein: We do treat the nodes if the axilla is positive. We do very few axillary samplings in N-O patients. I am ashamed to say it, but perhaps it may prove to be right.

Kurtz (Seattle): In Seattle with node-positive patients, they do not get the axilla treated but they do get their supraclavicular and internal mammary nodes treated as a rule when they get chemotherapy. Usually the chemotherapy is given concomitantly with the radiotherapy.

Montague: We do the axillary dissection, and if the nodes are positive we would treat the internal mammary and supraclavicula in the region of the breast. If they have 1–3 positive nodes they get radiation first and then go onto a FAC program. If they have 4 or more positive nodes, they get the FAC first. After three courses, they get irradiated, then they go back to FAC.

Richardson (Seattle): I'd like to ask a question of Dr. *Prosnitz* and perhaps a comment by Dr. *Montague*. Sometimes I hear that there seems to be a greater recurrence locally with using electron beam rather than the iridium implant. I wonder if I could have a comment.

Prosnitz (New Haven): I personally am not convinced that that is the case. I think if you talked to Dr. *Hellman* of Boston, you'd learn that he's not convinced of that. Maybe it depends on what day you talk to him. Actually the patients in the Boston group who got the implant were treated later on, so the figures are a bit skewed by the fact that there is a shorter follow-up in the implant patients. I don't think there's a difference, and it's hard to imagine radiobiologically why there should be much of a difference between a given dose of electron beam and a given dose of implant.

Montague: I could't agree more. In fact, in the last article that the Boston group published, you will see that they have softened very much their recommendation of an isotopic implant. It's not being done in everybody, and I think that's the way it should be.

Buthune (Nova Scotia): Much of the discussion today seems to revolve around whether we are going to treat or not treat axillary nodes by radiotherapy. I'm getting the impression now that radiotherapists are wondering whether axillary radiotherapy is necessary or not. I would like to ask Dr. *Clark* to comment on his patients that didn't receive any radiotherapy and seemed to do pretty well, what other patients there were, what clinical stage they were and what the actual survival was. As surgeons I think we are more interested in survival than we are in the percentage of local recurrence.

Clark: Their survival is the same, and they started off as being a group of patients with minimal disease, but then later on the majority of them, I think, just did not receive, as a policy, any further treatment. We have added to that number, and we intend to follow these people with interest.

Ghossein: I think it is important to realize that a good number of those patients will lose their breasts because of local recurrence. I believe the recurrence rate in the breast is about 25%. So you are going to be obliged to do another surgical procedure which will make the woman lose her breast. That could have been avoided by giving moderate doses of radiations, and that's crucial, I think.

Montague: I think all of us who do a substantial amount of breast irradiation realize that there is a subset of the patient population that probably will not require irradiation of the breast. We have to direct some attention to establishing who is in that subset. Is it a single focus of tubular carcinoma, is it a very well-differentiated lesion, a very small circumscribed focally invasive carcinoma, we really don't know. I think anyone of us can guess, but we don't have any scientific backup. Dr. *Clark's* 25% failure in the breast is repetitious because somebody else reported 25% failure in the breast with noninvasive intraductal disease excised only. There was a 25% failure 20 years ago when noninvasive intraductal disease was excised. So again we see a quarter of the patients will require further treatment. The question you have to ask yourself is, 'Is this acceptable to you?' If it's acceptable to you, then you may learn something from your experience in following these patients. But there is a better way to learn, and although the NSAPP is not very popular in most radiotherapy worlds (and it's not very popular with me sometimes either), I must say that they get the protocols done. Their recent protocol gives an axillary dissection in everybody, a segmental resection in one third of the patients, a segmental and breast irradiation only in the other third, and a modified radical in the third arm. But it's only by means of putting in 2,000 or 3,000 patients and then subsequently breaking them down pathologically and looking at various subsets that we have any hope of learning which subset of the patient population requires nothing other than segmental and axillary dissection or even forget the axillary dissection and just do the segmental. It's the control study, I think, even though I agree with Dr. *Clark,* which is very difficult to do. It's only under that kind of control that we really can learn about the biological behavior of the disease.

Prosnitz: I would like to second what Dr. *Montague* has just said in reference to what one is going to accept as a failure rate, and secondly with respect to her comments about randomized trials. I think that randomized trials are still critical for solving many issues, not solving all issues, but certainly many issues. I would like to comment on what Dr. *Clark* has said and what has been reported with the implication being that local recurrence managed by excising the lesion only or if one has already irradiated the breast that local recurrence is not going to impact the prime survival. That strikes me in the long run as being highly unlikely. I realize that their data may be showing that initially, but we are measuring survival now from the time of diagnosis, and we are talking about a group of local recurrences, many of which have occurred many years after diagnosis. I suspect that if we follow these patients long enough that it is going to impact. It's asking a lot of us to believe that if you allow a patient to fail locally from any kind of cancer, other than skin cancer, that that doesn't subject them to some kind of survival risk. I was in San Francisco 6 months ago for a Hodgkin's Symposium, and this very issue arose. Could you allow a patient without risk to relapse? Would you treat all the early ones or moderately early ones with radiotherapy and let a whole group of them relapse because there was no risk to relapsing? Some people at the symposium took that position, but that's really not so. I think most of us would agree that you just can't be totally blasé about letting a patient fail locally without subjecting her to some increased mortality given enough follow-up time.

Lawton (Hampton, Iowa): If patients have a local excision, prior to irradiation, secondary to the excision of the breast, it has been reported that at least 25 % of these patients have cancer remaining in the breast, but 75 % are free of cancer after the local excision. I just wonder if maybe sometimes we are not curing a large number of patients with the local excision. This would add to your survival in the irradiated group.

Prosnitz: Yes, but that's what we do in all of medicine. If you take pneumococcal pneumonia and you don't treat it with anything, most of the patients don't die – they get better. Penicillin makes 99 % of them better, or whatever the number is. And that's what we do in everything, so, sure, maybe 75 % or 60 % or some number of them don't need the treatment. It depends on what the risk of the treatment is, what the morbidity of the treatment is, and it also depends on what failure rate you consider acceptable, as Dr. *Montague* has said a number of times.

Sacks (Santa Cruz, Calif.): Many radical mastectomies are being done in the United States for people who may not have any more disease in the breast. I think your question is really one that should not only come to the radiotherapists, but you should ask every single surgeon in the United States the same thing.

Levitt (Minneapolis): Not enough investigators are looking at the nuclear grade. There are more and more data coming out in the literature that point out that the differentiation in nuclear grade has almost as much influence on the prognosis as the size of the primary lesion and the number of axillary nodes. I would also like to ask Dr. *Clark* if he would clarify the present philosophy of treatment at Princess Margaret. As I understood his talk, there are going to be some modifications in the way they treat breast cancer patients from what they have done in the past.

Clark: I think we do agree that what we are doing in radiation therapy at the present time is trying to preserve the breast; we are not influencing survival, so we will continue to give radiation to the breast alone. We already know that axillary dissections seem to add nothing in terms of survival as far as the patient is concerned. I think the same thing applies to the internal mammary nodes. We are one of the few groups looking at the internal mammary nodes at all. We are using the axillary dissection now as a prognostic factor, and we are using internal mammary scanning as a prognostic factor, too, and that will influence our use of adjuvant therapy subsequently.

Cantril: We have heard at this symposium probably two thirds of the available clinical data regarding radiation therapy for breast cancer available in the free world, I would guess, in one presentation or another. The presentations have been impressive. I've been in the field about 15 years and have been waiting from somebody to summarize the subject for me in such a concise form. The symposium proceedings published as volume 17 of *Frontiers in Radiation Therapy and Oncology* will be a marvelous contribution to the entire radiotherapy and oncological community.

Front. Radiat. Ther. Onc., vol. 17, pp. 115–123 (Karger, Basel 1983)

Adjuvant Chemotherapy and Hormonal Therapy for Operable Breast Cancer

David R. Minor

Departments of Medical Oncology, Marshall Hale Hospital and Children's Hospital, San Francisco, Calif., USA

Breast cancer remains the leading cause of death due to cancer in women. In 1982, over 100,000 women in America will develop breast cancer, and although the vast majority of these women will present with operable lesions, the past experience shows that over half of these women may relapse and die of their disease. Thus, our primary concern must be to design a treatment strategy that will maximize a woman's chance for survival and cure.

During the 1950s and 1960s vigorous attempts were made to increase survival of women with breast cancer through more vigorous local therapy with supraradical mastectomies and extensive postoperative radiation therapy. With a few expections, these attempts failed to increase survival, and current thinking on surgery and radiation therapy for breast cancer focuses on defining local therapies that will give both local control and acceptable cosmetic results.

The overwhelming majority of women who die of breast cancer die not because of failure of local control, but because at the time they present with a seemingly localized tumor in the breast, they already have microscopic deposits of tumor cells in distant organs or micrometastases. These micrometastases each contain from a few hundred to 10 million tumor cells and are undetectable by current X-rays or scans. Thus, for these women breast cancer is a systemic disease, and improvement in their survival depends on effective systemic therapy which will eradicate the micrometastases. The existence of distant micrometastases is an established experimental fact in laboratory animals and an established clinical fact for women with breast cancer. Without systemic therapy 75% of women with tumors metastatic to the axillary lymph nodes will develop distant metastases due to the growth of micrometastases present at the time of initial diagnosis. For women without axillary metastases, 25% have micrometastases present at initial diagnosis and will eventually also develop distant metastases.

In the 1970s we have seen the development of effective systemic therapy for operable breast cancer. This development is the most important advance in the treatment of breast cancer in this century. Until now, all any therapy, whether radiation or surgery, could achieve was only local control of the disease, and thus failed for the majority of women for whom breast cancer is a systemic illness. With the advent of effective systemic therapy, including chemotherapy and in some cases endocrine therapy, for the first time in decades we should begin to see a decline in mortality rates from breast cancer.

Armed with the understanding that treatment failure was due to micrometastases and the availability of chemotherapy drugs that were effective in advanced breast cancer, two large clinical trials were begun in the early 1970s to determine whether systemic chemotherapy, when added to standard surgical therapy, would be beneficial.

The best known of these trials, that of *Bonadonna* et al. [1, 13], was designed to determine whether adjuvant chemotherapy, consisting of a 1-year course of cyclophosphomide, methotrexate, and 5-fluorouracil, would alter the rates of relapse-free survival and overall survival in patients with metastatic deposits in axillary lymph nodes. In order to do this, 386 patients over a 3-year period were randomly allocated to receive either chemotherapy or no further therapy after surgery.

The answer was that chemotherapy significantly and rather dramatically improved patient survival. The relapse-free survival at 5 years increased from 44.6 to 59.5%, a 33% increase. As virtually all women who relapse will die of their disease, the eventual survival difference may be in this range with prolonged follow-up. With 5 years of follow-up, adjuvant cytoxan, methotrexate, and 5-fluorouracil increased overall survival from 66.2 to 78.4%, a 18% increase. Both these differences were statistically significant. Overall the study of *Bonadonna and Valagussa* [1] stands as a landmark success indicating for the first time that multidrug chemotherapy could increase survival for women with operable breast cancer. In analyzing this study it is important to observe which groups showed the most benefit. Women with 1 to 3 axillary lymph node appeared to benefit more than women who had 4 or more lymph nodes involved, as that group still had a high relapse rate. Premenopausal women showed considerable benefit, with 5-year relapse-free survival increased from 43 to 66%, a 52% increase in survival. For postmenopausal women, there was only a slight benefit to receiving chemotherapy which was not statistically significant. The detractors of chemotherapy looked at the failure of chemotherapy to help postmenopausal women and the beneficial effect in premenopausal women and claimed that the apparent benefit in premenopausal women of the chemotherapy drugs was because cytoxan had caused the patients to have ovarian failure and thereby indirectly forestalled relapse rather than having a direct tumoricidal effect on the micrometastases. This theory was based on earlier studies in the 1950s which had demonstrated that prophylactic oophorectomy would delay relapse in premenopausal women without resulting in long-term survival benefit.

There are, however, four reasons why systemic chemotherapy in premenopausal women was almost certainly effective because of a tumoricidal effect on micrometastases rather than due to any endocrine effects of chemotherapy. First, the 5-year follow-up of the studies of *Bonadonna* et al. [13] and *Fisher* et al. [7] shows that chemotherapy is effective in prolonging overall survival whereas prophylactic oophorectomy does not prolong overall survival. Second, there was no correlation in the study of *Bonadonna* et al. [13] between drug-induced amenorrhea and relapse-free survival, as would be expected if the benefit was due to drug-induced amenorrhea. Third, *Fisher* et al. [7] found that chemotherapy with melphalan showed the most beneficial for women aged 30–39 years while drug-induced menstrual changes were most apparent in women aged 40–49 years. The fourth and final argument against chemotherapy being effective due to endocrine effects comes from recent studies from Case Western and University of Texas, the study of *Hubay* et al. [10], which show that the addition of an endocrine therapy, tamoxifen, to chemotherapy may result in additional improvement in both pre- and postmenopausal patients.

The second major controlled randomized study to demonstrate the advantage of systemic chemotherapy in patients with operable breast cancer is that of the National Surgical Adjuvant Breast Protocol No. 5, the study of *Fisher* et al. [7]. The patients were randomly allocated to therapy with oral melphalan every 6 weeks for 2 years or to placebo. Patients who received melphalan had an increased disease-free survival that was statistically significant. In a pattern similar to the study by *Bonadonna* the benefit was most apparent in premenopausal women with metastases to 1, 2, or 3 lymph nodes.

Table I. Studies showing the efficacy of adjuvant chemotherapy in postmenopausal patients

Study group	Year of study beginning	Number of patients
Bonadonna and Valagussa [1]	1973	386
M. D. Anderson [2]	1974	222
Northwestern [3]	1975	173
Cooper et al. [4]	1968	73
COG [5]	1974	272
NSABP [7]	1972	1,848
SWOG [8]	1977	750
CALGB [9]	1975	376
Nissen-Meyer [12]	1965	1,136

The results of these initial trials [7, 13] failed to demonstrate statistically significant improvement in survival for postmenopausal women. This led to the continuing controversy over whether systemic adjuvant chemotherapy is indicated for postmenopausal women with operable breast cancer. Although unfortunately the mentioned authors and others in charge of designing clinical trials stopped randomizing postmenopausal women to placebo or control arms before they had proved the chemotherapy was beneficial, there is now abundant evidence that chemotherapy is effective from several new studies (table I).

The first study [1] is a retrospective analysis of *Bonadonna's* data looking at the dose-response curve for adjuvant chemotherapy. In carrying out this study the authors gave reduced doses of chemotherapy to women over 65 years of age in the mistaken belief that elderly patients tolerate chemotherapy less well than younger patients. Thus, many of this postmenopausal patients received very low doses of chemotherapy.

When they retrospectively reviewed their data on their premenopausal patients, they saw the best survival results in patients who received dose levels of 100–85 % or more of their planned chemotherapy regimen. This really is the same as seen with radiation therapy. We get better results giving 6,000 rad than giving 4,000 rad. For their postmenopausal patients who received full doses of chemotherapy they also saw good results with much fewer relapses than expected, although these data based on a small number of patients.

The second study to show improvement in survival for postmenopausal patients with adjuvant chemotherapy was the National Surgical Adjuvant Breast Protocol [7] studies No. 7 and 8. Although the authors found no improvement with single-drug chemotherapy, protocols No. 7 and 8, using 2- or 3-drug chemotherapy showed statistically significantly improved survival over historical controls. Although historical controls were used, these studies included 1,800 patients and had results similar to those of *Bonadonna and Valagussa* [1] or the 24,000 patients studied by the American College of Surgeons National Survey in 1977 [10]. Other studies which show the benefit of chemotherapy in postmenopausal women include the results of *Cooper* et al. [4], the developers of multidrug chemotherapy, who showed survival twice that of historical controls in 73 women followed for 5 years.

The Southwestern Oncology Group, in a study of 750 women [8], showed a 5-drug chemotherapy regimen to be superior to single-drug chemotherapy. Statistically significant differences for disease-free survival and overall survival were seen for both pre- and postmenopausal women. The Cancer and Acute Leukemia Group B, *CALGB*, studying 376 women comparing a 5-drug with a 3-drug regimen [9] showed a statistically significant prolongation in disease-free survival for postmenopausal women who received a 5-drug adjuvant chemotherapy regimen. The Central Oncology Group, *COG*, studied 272 patients with a 4-drug versus a 1-drug program and found superiority in the disease-free interval and overall survival for postmenopausal women receiving the 4-drug regimen [5]. All three of these controlled cooperative group studies showed superior results for 4- or 5-drug chemotherapy for postmenopausal women. Unless one proposes that the single-drug therapy given the control groups in these trials was detrimental, the conclusion that multiple-drug therapy is beneficial for postmenopausal women appears inescapable.

Confirmation of this benefit is also present in the data from M. D. Anderson, the study by *Buzdar* et al. [2], where adjuvant chemotherapy including doxorubinicin has been used since 1974. In treating 153 patients with stage II disease, their disease-free 5-year survival was 73% for premenopausal and 71% for postmenopausal patients, similar to the 76 achieved by *Bonadonna* et al. [13] for the selected group that tolerated full-dose chemotherapy. Thus, multiple studies document the effectiveness of adjuvant chemotherapy for postmenopausal women provided three or more drugs are given and full doses are administered.

The next important question is whether a systemic hormonal manipulation can improve survival for women with breast cancer. Although oophorectomy was first suggested over 90 years ago as possible adjuvant treatment with mastectomy, subsequently there have been few properly controlled clinical trials of endocrine therapy. Some trials in the 1950s seemed to indicate that surgical oophorectomy would delay relapse without any overall benefit on survival. At least one study of adjuvant ovarian irradiation and long-term prednisone, however, seemed to show some survival benefit for postmenopausal women.

With the advent of the estrogen receptor assay in the 1970s, however, we can now for the first time direct adjuvant endocrine manipulations towards those patients whose tumors would be expected to respond, patients who are estrogen receptor positive. In another landmark study, *Fisher* et al. [6] compared adjuvant 2-drug chemotherapy, melphalan and 5-fluorouracil, with the same 2-drug chemotherapy regimen with the addition of tamoxifen, a nontoxic antiestrogen compound. They were able to correlate the effectiveness of tamoxifen with the patients' estrogen receptor assay. In patients older than 50 years there was a 48 % reduction in relapse rate which was most pronounced in women with high estrogen receptor assay titers. A similar study form San Antonio and Case Western, the study by *Hubay* et al. [10], also showed benefit from adding tamoxifen to adjuvant chemotherapy. Since the follow-up on these studies is short, we do not yet know whether tamoxifen will prolong survival as well as delay relapse. Since the drug is virtually nontoxic, however, it may be useful in this setting, even if all it does is delay the onset of disseminated disease, so for the moment adjuvant tamoxifen would seem indicated in post-menopausal women with estrogen receptor positive tumors.

Patients who do not have axillary node metastases at presentation have a generally good prognosis, yet 25 % will eventually develop metastases and die from their disease. Before entertaining consideration of systemic therapy in this group, the determination of high-risk patients within this group is important. The tumor size itself is relatively unimportant. The cure rate for 5-cm tumors in 60 %, whereas for 1-cm tumors it is 70 %. A crucial prognostic factor for node-negative patients, however, is the estrogen receptor assay, for several studies showing that estrogen receptor negative patients, especially if premenopausal, have a poor prognosis. In another study by *Valagussa* et al. [14] of 464 node-negative patients who did not receive any adjuvant systemic therapy, the 5-year relapse-free survival for estrogen receptor assay negative premenopausal patients was only 38 %. Clearly for this group local therapy is not enough. Ongoing trials of adjuvant chemotherapy for this group have been started by *Bonadonna* and

Fisher. Until they are finished, routine adjuvant therapy cannot be recommended for this group, but should be considered on an individual basis.

Now that systemic chemotherapy and endocrine therapy, with the addition of tamoxifen, affords us means of systemic control of the disease, meticulous attention to details in achieving local control may be more important than ever. In the study of *Bonadonna* et al. [13], 84 patients treated with chemotherapy relapsed, and 21 % of those relapses were local or regional only.

Although the importance of giving full doses of chemotherapy early and other considerations discourage us from recommending postoperative radiation therapy prior to chemotherapy, the possibility of decreasing local relapse by giving radiation therapy after chemotherapy is largely unexplored, as is the question of appropriate timing of therapy for women who have radiation therapy rather than surgery as their primary local treatment modality.

To summarize our current management recommendations: all patients should have adequate therapy for local control and biopsy of axillary lymph nodes to determine the prognosis as well as determination of estrogen and progesterone receptors on their primary tumors.

Premenopausal patients with positive axillary nodes should have combination chemotherapy and perhaps the addition of tamoxifen for estrogen receptor positive patients. Premenopausal patients without axillary node metastases with estrogen receptor assay negative have a poor prognosis, and if they are not enrolled in a clinical trial, they should be considered for chemotherapy on an individual basis.

Postmenopausal patients with axillary metastases should have combination chemotherapy with tamoxifen added if the estrogen receptor assay is positive. Postmenopausal patients without axillary node metastases have a generally good prognosis, and adjuvant therapy would not seem to be indicated in this situation.

In the future we may expect more studies to determine the utility of early systemic therapy for patients without axillary node metastases and further work on drug schedules and combinations, so that all patients may tolerate 'full doses' and achieve the benefit that goes along with that. In the future further 'in vitro' tests will be performed on the primary tumor to determine what drugs to use. The estrogen receptor assay tells us whether to use tamoxifen, soon other in vitro assays will tell us whether or not to use cyclophosphamide or methotrexate or doxorubinicin. These assays may or may not be similar to the clonigenic assay developed at the University of Arizona.

The future for the therapy of breast cancer looks because after a century of preoccupation with radical mastectomy and local control, we have recognized breast cancer for the systemic disease that it is and have developed systemic therapies for it. All patients with breast cancer should be seen by a medical oncologist who has the experience to determine whether chemotherapy is needed and the art and skill to administer it, if needed, in adequate doses to prevent disease recurrence.

References

1   Bonadonna, G.; Valagussa, P.: Dose-response effect of adjuvant chemotherapy in breast cancer. New Engl. J. Med. *304:* 10–15 (1981).

2   Buzdar, A. U.; Blumenschein, G. R.; Hortobagy, G. N., et al.: Adjuvant chemotherapy with fluorouracil, doxorubinicin, and cyclophosphamide (FAC) in stage II or III breast cancer. 5-year results; in Jones, Salmon, Adjuvant therapy of cancer, vol. 3 (Grune & Stratton, New York 1981).

3   Caprini, J. A.; Oveido, M. A.; Cunningham, M. P., et al.: Adjuvant chemotherapy for stage II and III breast carcinoma. J. Am. med. Ass. *244:* 243–246 (1980).

4   Cooper, R. G.; Holland, J. F.; Gildewell, O.: Adjuvant chemotherapy of breast cancer. Cancer *44:* 793–798 (1979).

5   Davis, H. L.; Metter, G. E.; Ramirez, G., et al.: Adjuvant trial of 1-phenylalanine mustard (1-PAM) vs. cyclophosphamide (C), methotrexate (M), 5-fluorouracil (F) and vincristine (V) – CMFV – following mastectomy for operable breast cancer. Proc. AACR ASCO *22:* 426 (1981).

6   Fisher, B.; Redmond, C.; Brown, A., et al.: Treatment of primary breast cancer with chemotherapy and tamoxifen. New Engl. J. Med. *305:* 1–6 (1981).

7   Fisher, B.; Redmons, C.; Fisher, E. R.: The contribution of recent NSABP clinical trials of primary breast cancer therapy to an understanding of tumor biology. An overview of findings. Cancer *46:* 1009–1025 (1980).

8   Glucksberg, H.; Rivkin, S.; Rasmussen, S.: Adjuvant chemotherapy for operable breast cancer with positive axillary nodes. Proc. AACR ASCO *22:* 426 (1981).

9   Holland, J. F.; Torney, D.; Weinber, V., et al.: Adjuvant chemotherapy for breast cancer with 3 or 5 drugs – CMF vs. CMFVP. Proc. AACR ASCO *22:* 386 (1981).

10 Hubay, C. A.; Pearson, O. H.; Marshall, J. S., et al.: Antiestrogen, cytotoxic chemotherapy, and bacillus Calmette-Guérin vaccination in stage II breast cancer. A preliminary report. Surgery *87:* 494–501 (1980).

11 Nemoto, T.; Vana, J.; Bedwan, R. N., et al.: Management and survival of female breast cancer. Results of a national survey by the American College of Surgeons. Cancer *45:* 2917–2924 (1980).

12 Nissen-Meyer, R.: One short chemotherapy course in primary breast cancer: 12 year follow-up in series 1 of the Scandinavian adjuvant chemotherapy study groups; in Jones, Salmon, Adjuvant therapy of cancer, vol. 2 (Grune & Stratton, New York 1979).

13 Rossi, A.; Bonadonna, G.; Valagussa, P., et al.: Multimodal treatment in operable breast cancer. Results of a national survey by the American College of Surgeons. Cancer *45:* 2917–2924 (1980).
14 Valagussa, P.; DiFrouso, G.; Bignomi, P., et al.: Prognostic importance of estrogen receptors (ER) to select node negative (N−) patients for adjuvant chemotherapy. Proc. AACR ASCO *22:* 447 (1981).

D. R. Minor, MD, Director of Medical Oncology, Marshall Hale Hospital, San Francisco, CA 94118 (USA)

Front. Radiat. Ther. Onc., vol. 17, pp. 124–130 (Karger, Basel 1983)

Selection and Follow-Up of Patients for Conservation Surgery and Irradiation

Eleanor D. Montague, David D. Paulus, Sylvia R. Schell

Division of Radiotherapy, University of Texas, M.D. Anderson Hospital and Tumor Institute at Houston, Houston, Tex., USA

Recent reports have indicated that clinically favorable breast cancer can be successfully treated by excision of gross tumor in the breast and axilla followed by radiation therapy of moderate dose [2, 5, 7]. We have previously emphasized the importance of creating a field of treatment in which only subclinical disease exists, so that 4,500–5,000 rad tumor dose delivered to the breast and regional lymphatics, plus a boost of 1,000 rad to the tumor site, can be expected to control 95 % of the treated areas [5]. To achieve this high local control it is important for a team consisting of a diagnostic radiologist, surgeon, radiotherapist, and pathologist to engage in the selection of patients, and for the surgeon and radiotherapist to treat and follow all patients. This paper reviews the selection and follow-up of patients to be treated conservatively, placing particular interest on the use of mammography, either with film or xeroradiographic techniques.

Selection of Patients

Patients are clinically suitable for conservative surgery and irradiation if the primary tumor-bearing area is equal to or less than 4 cm, and in a breast ample enough for a good cosmetic result after excision of the tumor. Initially, only patients with a clinically negative axilla were treated, but since 1974, when a dissection of the lateral axilla was added, the presence of small mobile low axillary lymph nodes has not precluded conservative treatment. Pretreatment mammography is done on every patient to determine accurately (a) the size and position of the tumor in unbiopsied patients (b) the presence of multiple suspicious areas (c) the possibility of residual tumor or microcalcifications in previously biopsied patients, indicating the need for re-excision or larger boost dose, and (d) the status of the opposite breast.

Size and Position

Tumor measurement is more accurate on mammograms than on clinical examination, and therefore the mammogram measurement is the one generally used. Mammography can be used to map the boost field or the implant. The surgeon can also aid accuracy by placing clips to outline the margins of excision.

Multiple Sites

If the mammogram discloses multiple abnormal areas of relatively circumscribed disease with an aggregate diameter less than 4 cm, conservative surgery can be performed with good cosmetic result. However, when the suspicious sites in the breast are widespread, the patient is considered unsuitable for conservative surgery. Figure 1 demonstrates the situation in a 47-year-old woman whose excision biopsy revealed a 3×2 cm mass in the lower outer quadrant of the left breast 1 week prior to referral. The incision was healed and clinical examination was negative. However, she was unsuitable for conservation surgery because of at least three other sizable sites of disease.

Residual Tumor

As reported by *Gefter* et al. [1], mammograms can show gross residual tumor that must either be removed surgically or receive a higher dose of irradiation. Because of our previous report indicating that the incidence of late complications increases with dose and duration of follow-up, and a recurrence rate that is higher in patients who have had biopsy prior to referral (table I), a re-excision of the primary site is performed whenever possible, in addition to the dissection of the lateral axilla [5, 6]. If a re-excision is not possible because of local tissue disturbance, a boost of 1,500–2,000 rad tumor dose is given with an implant.

Opposite Breast

Pretreatment mammography of the contralateral breast is most important, in order to determine the presence of suspicious occult abnormalities

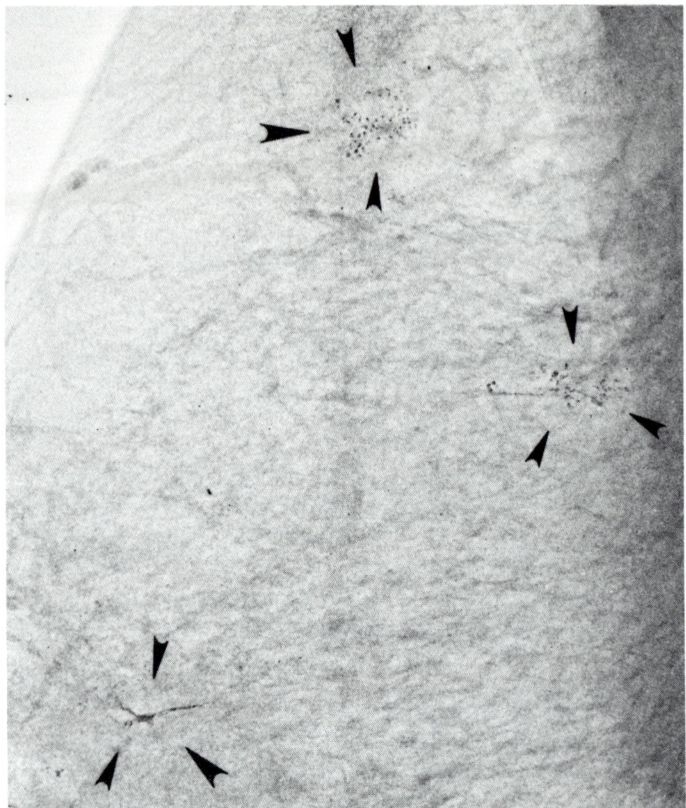

Fig. 1. Patient, age 47, seen in March 1980, with a 1 month's history of a 3 × 2 cm mass in the lower outer quadrant of the left breast. The mass was excised prior to referral and demonstrated infiltrating carcinoma of the breast. No other masses were palpated in the breast. The xeromammogram demonstrated three other sites suspicious for disease. The patient was not considered suitable for conservation surgery and irradiation, and had a left modified radical mastectomy.

Examination of the specimen demonstrated a 3.0 cm carcinoma immediately underlying the nipple and a 1-cm carcinoma in the upper outer quadrant of the breast. In addition, there were multiple areas of intraductal carcinoma, the largest one measuring 1.5 cm. The patient had postoperative irradiation to the regional lymphatics and chest wall (5,500 rad given dose/5 weeks with electrons) and remains well as of February 1982.

Table I. Local recurrence in patients treated with conservation surgery and irradiation (1955–1979; analysis January 1982)

MDAH excision		Excision biopsy prior to referral	
n	%	n	%
4/140	2.9	10/123	8.1

that can be biopsied at the same time. If these prove malignant, bilateral irradiation can be planned, determined by stage of disease and location of tumor in the breast.

Follow-Up of Patients

All patients treated with conservation surgery and irradiation should be followed by the radiotherapist and the surgeon. A posttreatment baseline mammogram of the treated breast is obtained within 6 months of treatment. Thereafter, annual bilateral mammograms are obtained. The diagnostic radiologist must always be made aware of prior irradiation of the breast, since the secondary skin and stromal changes related to the radiation therapy may be confused with recurrent disease.

Clinical follow-up of patients is scheduled every 4 months for 3 years, every 6 months until the 6 year, and at yearly intervals thereafter. Thus far, six recurrences have been diagnosed clinically because of a small palpable mass, and eight recurrences were diagnosed on mammogram because of microcalcifications.

Figure 2 represents a xeromammogram showing microcalcifications in the upper outer quadrant of the left breast in a patient treated 8 years previously with irradiation after excisional biopsy; clinical examination remained negative. The patient had a modified radical mastectomy and remains free of disease. Figure 3 is the xeromammogram of a patient who had an excision of a primary tumor prior to referral. Unfortunately, no pretreatment xeromammogram was performed. Follow-up xeromammogram indicated multiple sites of microcalcifications, which were probably present initially and would have made the patient unsuitable for conservation surgery.

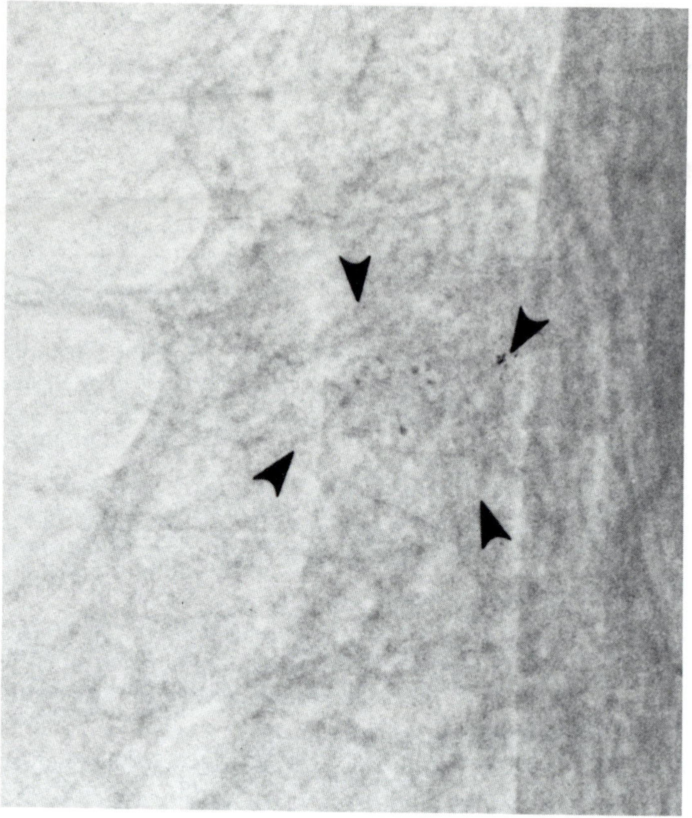

Fig. 2. Patient, age 65, seen in 1973, following an excision biopsy of an upper inner 2 × 3 cm carcinoma of the left breast prior to referral. A single histologically negative node in the axilla was also removed. The patient was treated in May and June 1973 with 5,000 rad tumor dose to the breast and regional lymphatic areas including the axilla, followed by 1,000 rad tumor dose in 5 days with 9-MeV electrons to a limited field covering the primary site. The patient remained well without roentgenographic or clinical evidence of recurrence until July 1981, when a xeromammogram showed suspicious-appearing calcifications in the upper outer quadrant of the left breast. A modified radical mastectomy was performed, which showed an infiltrating duct carcinoma measuring 1 × 1 cm in size, and negative nodes.

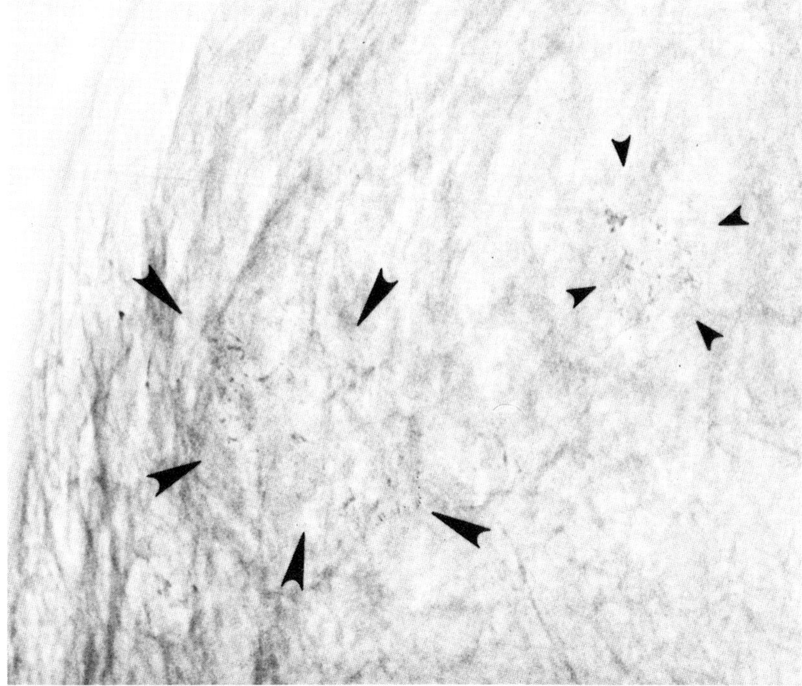

Fig. 3. Patient, age 59, seen in July 1976, following an excision biopsy of a 1.5 cm infiltrating duct carcinoma in the upper inner quadrant of the left breast. Unfortunately, a postbiopsy preirradiation xeromammogram was not obtained, nor had she had a mammogram prior to the biopsy. The patient was treated with radiation therapy, giving 5,000 rad tumor dose to the breast in addition to 1,000 rad tumor dose boost with 9-MeV electrons to the primary site. The axilla and peripheral lymphatics received 5,000 rad tumor dose in 5 weeks. Xeromammogram in July 1977 showed microcalcifications in the upper outer and central portions of the breast. A simple mastectomy was performed, which showed infiltrating carcinoma of the breast in the areas of high density on the specimen radiograph. The patient remains well and free of disease in February 1982.

Discussion

Prior reports from this institution have dealt with follow-up mammography in the irradiated breast. *Libshitz* et al. [3, 4] have reported that patients whose breast has received 5,000 rad tumor dose have skin thickening, which returns to normal appearance in 60 % of the patients in 2 years, in over 80 % in 3 years, and, by the end of 4 years, no abnormality can be detected in the skin [4]. In addition, dysplastic calcifications can develop following irradiation that are often irregular but may simulate secretory calcifications. These calcifications have occurred in 11% of patients who have undergone excision biopsy and radiation therapy, sometimes at the site of the cancer and only in the treated breast, perhaps due to necrotic tissue or other cellular debris [3]. It is important to recognize that benign calcifications can develop, so that they will not be confused with recurrent malignancy.

By means of close communication between all specialties concerned in the selection, treatment, and follow-up of patients with breast cancer treated with conservative surgery and irradiation, successful treatment can be achieved in over 90% of patients. Radiographic evaluation and follow-up of the affected breast is an important part of this combined approach.

References

1   Gefter, W.B.; Friedman, A.K.; Goodman, R.L.: The role of mammography in evaluating patients with early carcinoma of the breast for tylectomy and radiation therapy. Radiology *142:* 77–80 (1982).

2   Harris, J.R.; Botnick, L.; Bloomer, W.D.; Chaffey, J.T.; Hellman, S.: Primary radiation therapy for early breast cancer: the experience at the Joint Center for Radiation Therapy. Int. J. Radiat. Oncol. Biol. Phys. *7:* 1549–1552 (1981).

3   Libshitz, H.I.; Montague, E.D.; Paulus D.D.: Calcification and the therapeutically irradiated breast. Am. J. Roentg. *128:* 1021–1025 (1977).

4   Libshitz, H.I.; Montague, E.D.; Paulus, D.D.: Skin thickness in the therapeutically irradiated breast. Am. J. Roentg. *130:* 345–347 (1978).

5   Montague, E.D.; Gutierrez, A.E.; Barker, J.L.; Tapley, N. duV.; Fletcher, G.H.: Conservation surgery and irradiation for the treatment of favorable breast cancer. Cancer *43:* 1058–1061 (1979).

6   Spanos, W.J., Jr.; Montague, E.D.; Fletcher, G.H.: Late complications of radiation only for advanced breast cancer. Int. J. Radiat. Oncol. Biol. Phys. *6:* 1473–1476 (1980).

7   Veronesi, U.; Saccozzi, R.; Del Vecchio, M.; Banfi, A.; Clemente, C.; De Lena, M.; Gaiius, G.; Greco, M.; Luni, A.; Marubini, E.; Muscolino, G.; Rilke, F.; Salvadori, B.; Zecchini, A.; Zucali, R.: Comparing radical mastectomy with quadrantectomy, axillary dissection and radiotherapy in patients with small cancers of the breast. New Engl. J. Med. *305:* 6–11 (1981).

Prof. E.D. Montague, MD, Division of Radiotherapy, University of Texas, M.D. Anderson Hospital and Tumor Institute at Houston, Houston, TX 77030 (USA)

Front. Radiat. Ther. Onc., vol. 17, pp. 131–142 (Karger, Basel 1983)

Breast Irradiation and Future Risk of Carcinogenesis

S. H. Levitt, J. Mandel[1]

Department of Therapeutic Radiology, University of Minnesota Hospitals, and Department of Epidemiology, School of Public Health, University of Minnesota, Minneapolis, Minn., USA

Introduction

It is well accepted by most physicians and epidemiologists that irradiation to the breast area can be carcinogenic. This risk is dependent to a greater or lesser extent on a number of factors which include dose, number of exposures, age at exposure, ovarian function. It is a major concern for physicians who treat breast cancer with conservative surgery and radiation therapy because of the possibility of increased incidence of a second cancer in the contralateral breast, as well as in the treated breast.

The subject is complicated by the very diverse nature of the disease itself. It is difficult to ascertain whether recurrence in the breast itself is cancer secondary to irradiation, after a sufficient latent period, or whether it is disease which has remained inactive in that breast. Similarly, the development of a second primary cancer in the opposite breast is complicated by the fact that patients who do have unilateral breast cancer have an increased risk of developing a second cancer in the contralateral breast. The answer to the question raised by the title of this paper needs to address the epidemiologic factors involved in the development of breast cancer, and the natural occurrence of bilateral breast cancer (both simultaneous and consecutive). The evidence from the literature regarding the development of breast cancer secondary to irradiation will be examined and, insofar as possible, the present experience of consecutive breast cancer development

[1] The authors wish to acknowledge the editorial assistance of *Sarah Batzli,* and her help in the preparation of this manuscript.

in patients treated with surgery alone or surgery plus radiation therapy for their initial breast cancer will also be reviewed.

Epidemiologic Factors Involved in the
Development of Breast Cancer

The data on known risk factors for human breast cancer have been reviewed by *MacMahon* et al. [12] and by *Kelsey* [8]. 'Known risk factors' include the major predictors of risk, as age, geographic area of residence, age at first birth, certain indicators of ovarian activity, a history of benign breast disease, and a familial history of breast cancer. The study by *Kelsey* [8] on the epidemiology of human breast cancer pointed out that 1 in 14 women will develop breast cancer at some time in her life; however, these data need to be modified in view of the fact that there is an increasing number of women who have their first child at an older age, or who choose not to have children, and this relates to the association of breast cancer risk with nulliparity and older age at first birth. It is therefore likely that the incidence of breast cancer may become even higher in the future. There has also been an increasing incidence of breast cancer in women aged 45–74, and in black women. Thus, many factors enter into the epidemiology of breast cancer and must be considered.

A number of factors are worthy of note when one compares the risk of naturally occurring breast cancer to the risk of induced breast cancer in various populations treated in different ways. But most important among these considerations is the fact that diagnosis of fibrocystic breast will increase a woman's risk for breast cancer from two to four times. This increased risk has been found to persist for at least 30 years after the diagnosis of fibrocystic disease. Women in the upper socioeconomic classes have a higher tendency for both fibrocystic disease and breast cancer.

Women with breast cancer may have association with multiple primary cancers in other organs. For example, there is an increased relative risk of second primary cancer in the breast following ovarian cancer, ranging from approximately 1.5 to 4. Patients with endometrial cancer have an increased relative risk of 1.2 to 2.0 for a second primary breast cancer, but this usually occurs in women over the age of 60, and within 10 years after the diagnosis of the endometrial cancer. Women with breast cancer probably have a slightly elevated risk for endometrial cancer, but this is hard to evaluate.

There is also an increased incidence of cancer of the colon and rectum among breast cancer patients. Other associations which have been reported include acute myeloid leukemia, major salivary gland tumors, cancer of the buccal cavity and pharynx, meningioma, malignant melanoma of the eye, thyroid cancer, and soft tissue sarcoma. The genetic factors should probably also be considered. In general, it is reported that the genetic effect is greater in premenopausal cases than in postmenopausal cases, and is stronger in bilateral than in unilateral cases.

In summary, there are many factors which are involved in the epidemiology of breast cancer. Whether these factors would interact in the development of a second primary cancer in the contralateral breast must be considered in evaluating the effect of irradiation in the opposite breast and in evaluating the patients who develop cancer in the remaining, opposite breast.

Natural Occurrence of Bilateral Breast Cancer

One of the most important factors that must be considered in evaluating the carcinogenic effect of therapeutic irradiation is the incidence of bilateral breast cancers in patients who have not received radiation. There are several problems which complicate a study such as this: (1) the difficulty in differentiating metastatic disease from a second primary cancer; (2) the difficulty in evaluating the natural history of the disease; and (3) the difficulty in evaluating the effect of treatment, or the lack of treatment, on the natural history of the disease.

In the past, bilateral breast cancer was thought to be more common in patients in early stages of the disease because patients with more advanced disease did not live as long, and therefore could not develop the second disease. A classic study by *Robbins and Berg* [16] found that second breast cancers tended to arise in women who were less than 50 years of age at the time of the first mastectomy. The presence of multiple cancers in the first breast was associated with a particularly high risk. In contrast, if the first cancer was a well-differentiated carcinoma without metastases, the risk was almost halved.

The reported frequency of bilateral carcinoma varies from series to series, and estimates as high as 30 % have been reported in the literature. Some of these second cancers are carcinoma in situ, and, therefore, cannot be considered as accurate determinants of second carcinoma. The real rate of occurrence of bilateral disease therefore varies from 3 to 7% in all women in whom unilateral breast cancer develops.

In a paper by *Mueller and Ames* [14], the risk of bilaterality appears to have a rate of 0.8–1% per year in their population. The risk was reported to persist for approximately 15 years. In their series, the second primary cancer developed by the end of the 5th year in 75% of the patients. Thus, the overall risk of developing primary, nonsimultaneous breast cancer in the second breast is about 5 times greater for women who have previously had breast cancer than the risk in the general female population of developing a primary breast cancer.

Leis [10] has pointed out that factors which influence the incidence of subsequent primary breast cancers in the second breast include the length of follow-up, the prognostic status, the use of patient- versus breast-years, the variations in reporting standards and pathologic interpretations, and assiduity of the follow-up. He agreed with *Robbins and Berg* [16] that the risk of the patient developing cancer in the other breast was 5 times that of the general population. Those patients considered at high risk include patients whose cancer of the first breast carried a good prognosis for extended survival, and whose age and constitutional status did not exclude at least a 20-year normal life expectancy. Thus, patients under 50 years of age, in good health, with early cancers, which are noninvasive (or if invasive, of good prognostic type) were considered at high risk for developing subsequent cancer in the remaining breast. Also included are 'patients with a close family history of breast cancer, especially if bilateral and premenopausal, those whose cancers in the first breast were multicentric throughout the breast, and those who had evidence of precancerous mastopathy found on biopsy of the remaining breast.' In addition, patients with a P2 or DY parenchymal x-ray pattern of the remaining breast on the mammogram, or who had an abnormal thermogram, are included in the high-risk group.

Of major interest is the report by *Haagensen* [7] in which he noted that the incidence of carcinoma of the second breast when carcinoma of the first breast occurred under the age of 50 is 17 times the normal incidence, whereas the rate for women over 50 is 6 times the normal incidence. The average interval between the first and second primary breast carcinoma in his series was 10 years (the range being from 2 to 20 years). Thus, the relative incidence of 'naturally occurring' second breast cancer, that is non-consecutive, is one which must be kept in mind when evaluating the effect on the second breast of irradiation to the primary cancer in the first breast.

Carcinogenic Effect of Therapeutic Doses of Radiation in the Primary Treatment of Breast Cancer

A number of studies demonstrate an increased incidence of breast cancer secondary to the exposure to ionizing radiation. These findings are based on studies of Japanese patients exposed to the atomic bomb, patients with tuberculosis exposed to fluoroscopy in Massachusetts, patients with postpartum mastitis treated in Rochester, N.Y., and patients with benign breast disease treated in Sweden.

Boice et al. [2], in an article which comments on these studies, noted that the risk is greatest for persons exposed as adolescents, although exposure at all ages carries some risk. They further stated that the dose-response relationship is consistent with linearity in all studies, and that there is evidence of radiation risk at doses under 50 rads in atomic bomb survivors (0.5 Gy). To continue, 'Fractionation does not appear to diminish risk, nor does time since exposure (even after 45 years of observation). The interval between exposure and the clinical appearance of radiogenic breast cancer may be mediated by hormonal or other age-related factors but is unrelated to dose. Age-specific absolute risk estimates for all studies are remarkably similar. The best estimate of risk among American women exposed after age 20 is 6.6 excess cancers/10^4 WY-Gy (10^6 WY-rad). ... Analysis suggests that the risk is greatest for persons exposed as adolescents, although exposure at all ages carries some risk.'

It appears, then, that there is a risk of carcinogenesis associated with ionizing radiation, particularly in younger women. However, the exact amount of risk is somewhat controversial. A number of caveats about the risk of carcinogenesis should be made. First, although it has been stated that radiation is carcinogenic at any dose rate, it was noted [6] that, 'repair processes are known to exist at the cellular levels, and that low dose rates are less effective at producing cancer in animal species than high dose rates'. Despite this, the ICRP has recommended 'the use of the same linear relationship for all dose rates, hence in the analysis ... no account (was) taken of the dose rates. However, it should be recognized that not all scientists ... agree with the ICRP on this matter of dose rates'. A second caution with regard to assumptions about dose rate and carcinogenesis appeared in another paper [9]: there is 'some evidence that the risk from very high radiation doses, over 500 rads, may be less per rad than that from low-dose exposures'. Third, the reader should examine each study carefully for accuracy because inaccuracies in the performance of the studies may have led to an overestimation of the actual risk.

Space does not allow a thorough analysis of all the studies. Therefore, our comments will essentially be confined to those studies of patients treated therapeutically. However, it is likely that all the studies have flaws which would complicate analysis and evaluation. For example, one group reported on the interaction between radiation and other breast cancer risk factors in a group of 1,764 women who had been institutionalized for pulmonary tuberculosis between 1930 and 1954 [3]. The methodology for estimating the radiation dose to the breast included interviewing the physicians who had conducted the examination, questioning the patients who had been examined fluoroscopically, and coupling measurements of fluoroscopic exposure rates with absorbed dose Monte Carlo computation. The accuracy of the study must be questioned primarily because the patients were treated so many years ago (1930–1954), and they were not interviewed in person but by mail questionnaire. The questionnaire was sent to 1,146 women found alive as of July 1975, and 80 % responded. The women were asked whether they remembered the physicians' fluoroscopic procedure; specifically, whether she faced the physician or whether she had her back to him during fluoroscopy, or whether her position was varied or rotated. The authors pointed out that interpretations could not be made with any degree of certainty, that the results must be regarded as generating hypotheses and that they need to be confirmed by a larger series. These uncertainties were due to various problems: the small numbers involved, the unknown effect of the 22 % non-response rate for the questionnaire, the inability to obtain breast cancer risk factor information on most of the women who had died, the imprecision associated with retrospective deter-mination of fluoroscopic procedure, and associated radiation breast doses.

The Rochester study is an example of a major study related to the therapeutic use of radiation. The study included 606 patients, 571 of whom responded to a mail questionnaire. The patients were treated with orthovoltage radiation for post partum mastitis, and then matched to a control group (from another city) who were not treated with radiation for their postpartum mastitis. They were treated with x-rays of 175–200 Kv (no filtration noted). The radiation exposure doses in roentgens in air were known for each patient. From these data, doses to breast tissue were estimated to have ranged from 40 to 1,500 rads, with a mean of 377 rads.

We have pointed out the weaknesses of this study in previous publications [11]. Our findings were: 'The major weakness in the study was in the loss of follow-up of thirty per cent of the control groups with mastitis. By having approximately thirty per cent lost to follow-up, the inference one can draw regarding the breast cancer risk of acute postpartum mastitis without radiation treatment is weakened. The follow-up of the sisters of the control group also is unsatisfactory: of the 380 group C (control) females found, only 304 were asked for their sisters' name and address; of the 304 contacted, seventy-two failed to respond with information on sisters. Only 137 from the original 380 group C reported sisters. Of the siblings they yielded, only seventy-eight per cent (160) were involved in the study. The familial aggregation of breast cancer is a known risk factor. Perhaps among the uncontacted sisters there were many breast cancer subjects. Some group C females, in fact, knowing that their sister was ill may have refused to cooperate for concern about disturbing a sick sibling. The natural history and long term effects, if any, of acute postpartum mastitis must be better known in order to evaluate its possible risk for breast cancer. A more thorough follow-up of group C would have helped provide some information on this.'

We have further noted [11] that, 'There was no mention of a review of death certificates of New York State to ascertain whether any of group C females died. Through a review of death certificates, one may be able to identify subjects with a mention of breast cancer on the certificate. This would allow for a better estimate of the breast cancer experience among non-irradiated post-partum mastitis subjects. The same could be done for group D, their sibling controls. If breast cancer subjects were located through this review the Standard Mortality Ratios for these groups may be considerably increased and thereby possibly reduce the difference between them and the irradiated group.'

It is interesting to note that the Rochester patients did not show any age specificity for the development of breast cancer, which is in contrast with the Stockholm and the atomic bomb studies. This could indicate that the disease associated with pregnancy may very well be a predisposing factor to the development of breast cancer when patients are irradiated.

One additional factor which might have led to an increased incidence of breast cancer in the irradiated mastitis group is the fact that there was a statistically significant increase in chronic cystic mastitis in the irradiated group as compared to the nonirradiated group. It is well known that chronic cystic mastitis is a predisposing factor to an increased incidence of breast cancer.

The Swedish study [1] concerning breast cancer following irradiation of the breast for benign diseases reported an increased incidence of breast cancer in these patients 4 times that expected. Two additional facts were noted: (1) there was an age-dependent incidence, i.e., the cancer incidence rate depended on the age of the patient at the time of irradiation. There was a higher risk of developing breast cancer when the breasts were irradiated at lower ages. (2) The incidence of radiation in the nonirradiated breast was no more than expected.

The Swedish study reported on 1,115 women who were seen between 1927 and 1957 at the Radiumhemmet. They were treated with ionizing radiation for different nonneoplastic conditions of the breast, and had an average follow-up of 31.5 years. The clinical diagnosis of the irradiated lesions were fibroadenomatosis in 855 patients, acute mastitis in 120, and chronic mastitis in 49. There were 13 patients who were treated for unilateral breast hypertrophy.

Information on irradiation was obtained from the patients' records. In the vast majority of records, the relevant physical parameters were known. Treatments were usually given with x-rays of half value layer (HVL) between 0.9 and 1.8 mm of copper. In a few cases, x-rays of HVL between 0.1 and 0.3 mm of copper or gamma radiation with a teleradium unit were used. The treatments were given in one, two, or several series. In 85% of the treatments, the total radiation dose was given within 12 months; 11% of the treatments were within a period of more than 12 months but less than 60 months; and 4% had a treatment of 60 months.

Baral et al. [13] found that the latent period for the development of breast cancer increased with the increase in dose and also increased in patients who were treated over the 60-month period. The limitation of this study is the absence of a control group and the fact that many of the women were treated for fibroadenomatosis and chronic mastitis, which might predispose them to breast cancer. In addition, the treatment fractionation and protraction were unusual and cannot be compared to therapeutic techniques used for the treatment of breast cancer.

Present Experience of Consecutive Breast Cancer in Patients Treated with Surgery Alone or in Combination with Radiation Therapy for Their Initial Breast Cancer.

There are many articles in the literature which report on the use of radiation therapy in the treatment of primary breast cancer following lumpectomy or following only biopsy. The recurrence rates in these reports are uniformly favorable, and show a similar survival and recurrence rate to surgery alone. Many of these patients have been followed for years, some as long as 30 years. A major concern at this time is the possibility of developing a second primary cancer in the contralateral breast in these patients. Women who have been treated for breast cancer do have an increased risk of developing a second primary cancer. The question to be answered is what is the incidence of second primary cancer in the contralateral breast in patients treated with irradiation.

One of the more helpful studies is that of *Baral* et al. [1], in which the effect of radiation on benign breast disease was evaluated. Although they did find a significantly increased incidence of breast cancer in the irradiated breast, there was no essential difference in the observed versus the expected number of breast cancers in the nonirradiated breasts.

Peters [15] has verified that in her series of patients there has not been an increased incidence of breast cancer in the contralateral breast. A recent paper by *Clark* et al. [5] is a study of 680 patients (some of whom were treated by *Peters*) who were followed for 21 years, with an average survival follow up of 12 years. The incidence of consecutive disease in the contralateral breast was 2.2%, which is similar to the incidence reported in the literature.

A study at the Institut Gustave-Roussy [17], in which patients were randomized for mastectomy or tumorectomy plus radiation, shows a 2.25 and 3.5% incidence of contralateral breast cancer in the two respective groups. Over 50% of these patients have been followed for over 5 years. In a nonrandomized group of patients at this institution treated with tumor-ectomy plus radiation, or radiation alone, the incidence of patients with consecutive disease in the contralateral breast has been 3% with 40% of the patients followed for 5 years.

In a series of 896 patients treated at the Fondation Curie [4] between 1960 and 1975, 44 patients developed cancer in the contralateral breast. In a series of 233 cases treated with lumpectomy and irradiation over the same period, 9 developed contralateral tumors. This is an incidence of contrala-teral breast cancer of 3.8% in the lumpectomy plus radiation group, and 4.9% in the radiation alone group.

A paper of major interest is that of *Schell* et al.[18] which reported on a series of 2,076 patients with stage I and II breast cancer treated between 1947 and 1976 at the M.D. Anderson Hospital. They found consecutive breast cancer in the contralateral breast in 87 patients, 6 months after the diagnosis of cancer in the first breast. They noted that 58% of the second breast cancers were diagnosed in the first 5 years, and 83% were diagnosed in the first 10 years following treatment, although it has been generally accepted that a second primary cancer should be diagnosed only after an interval of 5 years. Of interest is their statement that from the techniques used, based on direct measurement in recent patients, the dose to the medial half of the contralateral breast ranged from 100 to 300 rads. The incidence of second breast primary cancer in patients treated by surgery only was 7.3%. The incidence in the overall group treated by radiation, including all types of radiation, was 3.4%.

Conclusions

Breast cancer in women is a complex disease with a number of predisposing and epidemiologic factors involved. There continues, and perhaps for some time there will continue, to be controversy over the most appropriate method of treatment. One of the most promising approaches to the treatment of breast cancer is the recent increased utilization of so-called 'lumpectomy' and primary radiation in the early stage I and II breast cancers. The survival results in these studies and the marked benefit insofar as the psychological effect on the patient have stimulated increased use of this approach and many women now insist that it be their treatment.

Complicating the problem of the disease itself and the best or most appropriate choice of treatment is the fact that radiation is a carcinogenic agent. There is no question that there is an increased incidence of breast cancer in individuals who are treated with radiation, particularly in the perimenarchial period, and in the ages of 10–19. Whether or not the doses of irradiation which are received by the average patient would lead to a significantly increased incidence of primary breast cancer in the contralateral breast is of major importance. The development of a second primary breast cancer could be a serious risk and a possible contraindication of the use of this approach.

Based on the evidence from the current clinical studies, there does not appear to be an increased risk of second primary in the contralateral breast. Caution must be taken, however, because many of the studies were only recently completed, and breast cancer following irradiation usually develops after approximately a 5- to 10-year interval from the time of radiation. It would appear from our review that the risk per rad may be overestimated, based on some of the problems in the studies of radiation breast carcinogenesis which we have already pointed out. Therefore, there is no apparent increased risk of second primary breast cancer from irradiation of the first primary breast cancer based on the currently available data. Further follow-up studies need to be undertaken and the question of treatment for the patient under age 25 is one which should be evaluated by the individual patient and physician.

References

1   Baral, E.; Larsson, L.-E.; Mattsson, B.: Breast cancer following irradiation of the breast. Cancer *40:* 2905–2910 (1977).
2   Boice, J.D.; Land, C.E.; Shore, R.E. et al.: Risk of breast cancer following low-dose radiation exposure. Radiology *131:* 589–597 (1979).
3   Boice, J.D.; Stone, B.J.: Interaction between radiation and other breast cancer risk factors; in Late biological effects of ionizing radiation, vol. 1. Proc. Symp., Vienna 1978, pp. 231–249 (IAEA, Vienna 1978).
4   Calle, R.: Personal communication.
5   Clark, R.M.; Wilkinson, R.H.; Mahoney, L.J. et al.: Breast cancer: a 21-year experience with conservative surgery and radiation. Int. J. Radiat. Oncol. Biol. Phys. (in press, 1982).
6   Dolphin, G.W.: Estimation of the risks of ionizing radiation. Archs Toxicol. *3:* Suppl., pp. 27–41 (1980).
7   Haagensen, C.D.: The natural history of breast carcinoma: in Haagensen Diseases of the breast (Saunders, Philadelphia 1971).
8   Kelsey, J.L.: A review of the epidemiology of human breast cancer. Epidemiol. Rev. *1:* 74–109 (1979).
9   Land, C.E.: Low-dose radiation – a cause of breast cancer? Cancer *46:* 868–873 (1980).
10 Loio, H.P.: Bilateral breast cancer. Surg. Clins N. Am. *21:* 459–465 (1978).
11 Levitt, S.H.; Potish, R.A.: The role of radiation therapy in the treatment of breast cancer: the use and abuse of clinical trials, statistics and unproven hypotheses. 1979 ASTR Presidential Address. Int. J. Radiat. Oncol. Biol. Phys. *6:* 791–798 (1980).
12 MacMahon, B.; Cole, P.; Brown, J.: Etiology of human breast cancer: a review. J. natn. Cancer Inst. *50:* 21–42 (1973).
13 Mettler, F.A.; Hempelmann, L.H.; Dutton, A.M. et al.: Breast neoplasms in women treated with x-rays for acute postpartum mastitis: a pilot study. J. natn. Cancer Inst. *43:* 803–811 (1969).
14 Mueller, C.B.; Ames, F.: Bilateral carcinoma of the breast: frequency and mortality. Can. J. Surg. *21:* 459–465 (1978).
15 Peters, V.: Personal communication.
16 Robbins, G.F.; Berg, J.W.: Bilateral primary breast cancers, a prospective clinicopathological study. Cancer *17:* 1501–1527 (1964).
17 Sarrazin, D.: Personal communication.

18 Schell, S.; Montague, E.D.; Spanos, W.J. et al.: Bilateral breast cancer (for future publication).

19 Shore, R.E.; Hempelmann, L.H.; Kowaluk, E. et al.: Breast neoplasms in women treated with x-rays for acute postpartum mastitis. J. natn. Cancer Inst. *59:* 813–822 (1977).

Prof. S.H. Levitt, MD, Department of Therapeutic Radiology, University of Minnesota Hospitals, Box 494 Mayo Memorial Building, 420 Delaware Street S.E., Minneapolis, MN 55455 (USA)

Front. Radiat. Ther. Onc., vol. 17, pp. 143–146 (Karger, Basel 1983)

Discussion

Dymott (San Francisco): Dr. *Levitt,* if you had a daughter age 30–35 with an operable breast cancer, would you have her treated by radiotherapy?

Levitt (Minneapolis): Yes. We all ought to keep in mind a number of things that came up in the program preceeding this discussion. I think it depends on the indications. I don't think that you can say that everybody ought to be treated this way. It depends on the stage, location, size of the breast, and a number of other factors, but if she were a reasonable candidate, then, yes, I would.

Dymott: Do we have any other questions from the floor?

Buthune (Nova Scotia): I am a practicing surgeon. I feel young women, perhaps 30–35, with a very bad family history, e.g. mother died of bilateral breast carcinoma at a young age and perhaps her sister, represent difficult situations, and I run into them quite frequently. What do I do about a follow-up of this particular young woman with respect to mammograms? We do know there is some increased risk in the overall group, a very small risk, but in this particular type of patient where all the risk factors are multiplied, it really is a concern. The other concern is equally related to the same type of patient, perhaps 32 or 35 years old, who has had a mastectomy for carcinoma. She has all the high family risk factors, she is young, she has had carcinoma, and the follow-up of this patient is also quite a concern, particularly because she is going to have mammograms for perhaps the next 35 years. I must admit I don't do it every year. I really don't know what to do, and I would like to hear your comments. The second question also is for Dr. *Levitt* and has to do with the subsequent development of cancer in the irradiated breast following lumpectomy. There is a Swedish study which seemed to show about a 4 time accelerated incidence of carcinoma in the irradiated breast.

Levitt: There is a risk with mammography, but I think it is really a minimal risk. By the way, I want to mention that the work you see here today and the work that I have done in the past has always been possible because of the cooperation of my colleagues in both biometry and epidemiology. At the present time we are in a study with Dr. *Mandel* of our epidemiology department of the actual risk per rad. I think it is estimated to be higher than it actually is. I think that the lady you are talking about has a very high risk factor, and I think she would need to have mammography. I would be uncomfortable with not following her because I think you are going to pick up an earlier cancer far sooner. At least in 50 % of the cases you can pick up an early cancer that you can't see or feel. Now as to the incidence of cancer in the treated breast, first of all I want to say that the Swedish study treated their patients in a very unusual manner. They were treated with orthovoltage radiations. Some of the patients were treated over a 5-year period. They had benign breast disease also. It is really difficult to translate that particular study into concern about the therapeutically treated breast. The doses were smaller, the equipment was different, and I think finally the recurrence rate in most of the series, almost every series that I've seen, had been with patients treated with conservation surgery and radiation has been similar to those with surgery alone. I do think that I am not concerned in that situation.

Lawton (Hampton, Iowa): I know that most of our therapies are double-edged swords, and I was wondering if someone would comment on the development of second cancers in those patients who are treated with chemotherapy. I know of quite a number of them, as I have collected a fair number myself. I wonder if you would comment on that.

Minor (San Francisco): I can comment on that. In *Bonnadonna's* study with a median follow-up of 5 years, he has seen no increased incidence of second malignancies in women treated with chemotherapy for breast cancer. Now that's not to deny that in patients with Hodgkin's disease, myeloma, ovarian carcinoma treated with long-time alkylating agents, there isn't an increased incidence of hematological malignancies. There most certainly is. But there may be other immunologic factors we don't understand about that. In the data on myeloma, and I think also the patients with ovarian carcinoma, if they're treated for 18 months or less with alkylating agents, they do not seem to have significantly increased risk of second malignancy or acute leukemia. There was one report in *ASCO* about 3 years ago of an old study from Philadelphia where 13 women got chlorambucil for 5 years as adjuvant therapy for breast cancer. 3 of them developed acute leukemia, so that it is a definite risk if the prolonged alkylating agents are used. With the currently recommended dosage regimens I don't think it is a significant problem. We don't have all the answers in terms of why, for example, patients with Hodgkin's disease do have such a high incidence of acute leukemia and other myeloproliferative problems following treatment. It may be something to do with their underlying disease.

Dymott: I'd like to comment, if I may. I think one point that you made is the fact that, and I think that's an important fact, that a lot of these patients have not been followed for a long enough time, and we are going to have to wait until 10, 15 or maybe even 20 years to see what really happens. There has been recently reported in the literature an experimental study in which mice treated with CMF developed an increased incidence of malignancy as opposed to control, and there are a number of articles in the literature relating to the development of second malignancies with chemotherapy. If you look through the literature, you'll find more and more of these, so I think they're toxic agents just like radiation, and I think we are going to have to keep our eyes open on all of these things including radiation.

Cantril (San Francisco): Dr. *Minor,* I was hoping you were going to clarify for me when radiation and chemotherapy are given simultaneously or sequentially and in what sequence in patients who are candidates for adjuvant chemotherapy. This seems to be a real bone of contention between our specialties. The second part of the question is as I understand *Bonnadonna's* 10-year data, the lines are coming together and that actually, at least as far as 10-year survival is concerned, it doesn't appear that there is an advantage for adjuvant chemotherapy.

Minor: In regard to the first question, I don't think that we really know the answer as to how to use both postoperative irradiation and chemotherapy. I think it's more desirable to probably give the chemotherapy first, or at least several months of the chemotherapy first, provided women have had some sort of mastectomy with removal of all gross disease. The theoretical basis for that is based upon the fact that tumor doubling size doubles about every month, and one or two doublings may dramatically increase the odds that micrometastases may eventually have enough cells to be resistant to chemotherapy. In animal models, adjuvant chemotherapy often works only if started early enough in the course of the disease. There are also some data from two studies that come to mind that point out the possible importance of early chemotherapy. One is a study I didn't mention earlier, a study from Sweden where approximately 700 women were all followed for at least 7–10 years. Half of them were randomized to 6 days of i.v. Cytoxan starting on the 3rd postoperative day. It seems like a very short and very small course of chemotherapy to expect any benefit, but 7 years down the line the survival for the patients getting the Cytoxan was 10% higher. That study would seem to indicate that early chemotherapy is important. Another study is that of *R. Cooper,* who did a historical control compared with patients that seemed to be fairly well matched for stage of disease. He compared, I believe, about 70 patients who received chemotherapy alone with 70 that received first postoperative radiation therapy for a couple of months, then chemotherapy. He found at the end of 7 years that of the patients that received chemotherapy alone, 75% were alive and free of disease. Of the ones that received radiation therapy followed by chemotherapy, only 25% were alive and free of disease. That would seem to indicate the sequence of holding off chemotherapy for a couple of months while radiation is being given is not proper, at least in patients that have had mastectomy. I think porbably the theoretically best way if the patient is stage II is to give the two modalities together, probably go ahead and give 1 year of chemotherapy first and then follow that with radiation. I think probably in that order you can get in full doses of both. Following extensive irradiation it can be difficult to get in a full course of chemotherapy for several reasons, radiation pneumonitis being one, another is that the irradiation will cause a transient lymphopenia so that the oncologist should be careful not to interpret this as being a reason to decrease his chemotherapy. In patients that are getting combined modality treatments, it is important for the oncologist to know he just should look at the granulocyte count rather than the total white count in determining his dose of chemotherapy. In answer to the second part of the question, *Bonnadonna's* study started in 1973 and he finished accruing patients in 1976, so that data we have are for an average of about 6 years. The curves do not seem to be coming together for premenopausal patients. There is still a very significant difference in survival. In fact, the differences in survival become more impressive with time. I'm talking about overall survival for the premenopausal patients. One of the questions was, How are the patients going to do survival-wise after they recur in the patients that received chemotherapy, and the patients that didn't seemed to have similar rapid demise following recurrence in both groups; they live about a year and a half no matter what treatment they get.

Ghossein (New York): To answer the *Cooper* study, I reviewed the radiotherapy group of the *Cooper* study. It's unfortunate that it was printed in *Cancer.* The groups are not at all similar. In fact, radiotherapy patients did not come to Dr. *Cooper* saying, 'Hey, by the way, you know I would like some radiotherapy and then give me some chemotherapy later on'. Compared to the group who received chemotherapy they are a dismal group of patients whoreceived radiotherapy initially, and that's why their survival is so dismal. The tumors were much larger, the tumors had invaded the skin, the tumors had more lymph node involvement, and that's why they were referred to the radiotherapist first and then to Dr. *Cooper* later. It is very infortunate that this study is often quoted. Now regarding the *Bonnadonna* study, in the latest publication from Dr. *Bonnadonna* (its senior author is *Rossi*) published in August,

1981,there is 0.04 in favor of the CMF group – a very minimal difference in survival between the two groups. There is a bias in the two groups between the control and the CMF group, and that bias is that there is an unequal proportion of young women in one of the two groups. If you remove from the study all patients 35 years or younger both from the control group and the CMF-treated group, you find an amazing thing – that neither the disease-free or the absolute survival is significant in the CMF-treated group compared to the control group. This means if you give CMF to women 36 years of age or older, the benefit both in disease-free survival or absolute survival doesn't exist compared to control. This letter was published, by the way, in the *British Medical Journal* after Dr. *Bonnadonna* did review these data; it's his data, by the way, and as you can see the total numbers are equal; it's about 170 in each arm, and the disease-free survival is 0.1 and the absolute survival, the total survival between the two groups, is 0.2, so they statistically are not significant. What it's telling us is for the very young age-group, yes, it is important to give systemic treatment because their prognosis with local treatment is dismal, but beyond the young age-group I am not so sure that CMF is showing any benefit all the way to the older age-group. It is very important to remember that we may be giving a lot of drugs to women beyond the age of 35 with no benefit.

Kathy Colman (San Francisco): Dr. *Levitt,* has there been any research done on children or young girls who had cardiac surgery and many chest X-rays in the developmental phase of the breast and then the later subsequent development of breast cancer? Has there been any correlation?

Levitt: No, there is a diagnostic radiological study that shows that women who had fluoroscopy for tuberculosis, and in those groups of patients in large enough numbers, they found and increased incidence of breast cancer. It seems to be related to younger women. The real risk seems to be between 10 and 13, right before the menses.

Unidentified: I could make a comment on that, *Kathy.* There are some data that come out of Boston Children's Hospital on 250 kV whole-lung irradiation for children with osteogenic sarcoma who survived. Girls in the prepubescent period of their lives had 100% development of bilateral breast cancer. There are only about 10 cases, and this is not published, I don't think, at least I don't know where, but it's from *D'Angio,* a personal communication to me some years ago.

Levitt: I just recently saw a young woman who had been overtreated for Hodgkin's disease and developed breast cancer in the area of overirradiation. I hope that I'm not leaving you with the impression that radiation is not a carcinogenic agent. What I'm saying is that the risk is not as high as it's supposed to be. But there still is a risk, and I don't think it's a risk in this particular situation with a breast cancer patient.

Front. Radiat. Ther. Onc., vol. 17, pp. 147–153 (Karger, Basel 1983)

Summary

Robert G. Parker

University of California, Los Angeles, USA

Ionizing radiations have been used in the treatment of humans afflicted by breast cancer since 2 months after the discovery of X-rays by Roentgen on November 6, 1895 (discovered November 5, 1895, reported November 6, 1895, and published November 8, 1895!). As noted by *J. Vaeth,* this original therapeutic use of radiations was only 1 year following the introduction of radical mastectomy by *Halsted* in Baltimore in 1894. Throughout the intervening years, classical radical mastectomy has remained the vigorously defended standard of treatment, primarily in the USA, while irradiation has been sporadically investigated as a primary treatment in England, Europe, Scandinavia and Canada.

Vaeth has listed the major contributors to the development of radiation therapy for operable cancer of the breast. A most remarkable experience is that of *Keynes,* who in 1924 started treating patients with interstitial radium following excision of the primary tumor. His results, reported in 1929, and his observations are comparable to today's studies.

Why have these accomplishments of *Keynes* and others, i. e. *Mustakallio, Peters, Lenz and Baclesse,* been ignored, particularly in the USA? The challenge has been summarized by *Vaeth:* 'Only a few hundred patients entered into earlier modified radical mastectomy series eased our surgical colleagues into accepting this less multilating procedure for their patients... How many thousands of cured and non-maimed patients must the radiation therapist of the world accumulate before tylectomy and radiation therapy take its place as an acceptable method of treatment of early carcinoma of the breast?'

Information has been presented in this symposium that for patients with 'operable' cancer of the breast, tylectomy followed by radiation

Table I. Tylectomy plus radiation therapy

Author	Number of patients	Primary tumor	Local control, %	Observation period, years
Prosnitz	293	st. I and II	92	2–12
Montague	232	≤ 4.0 cm	97.1	3–27
			(excision at MDAH)	
			91.9	
			(excision elsewhere)	
Ghossein	307	T1–2	92	> 5

therapy is as effective, measured by local tumor control and long-term (10 years) survival, functionally and cosmetically superior and less intimidating to the patient than total mastectomy in any form.

Control of the Primary Tumor

The frequency of local control of cancer in the breast varies with tumor size and other factors, but is unquestionably comparable to that resulting from mastectomy (table I). When the primary lesion is excised with histologically clear margins, the dose to the entire breast need not exceed 4,500–5,000 rad in 5–5½ weeks, delivered in daily increments of 180–200 rad, and the primary site may not require a 'boost' dose *(Montague)*. If a 'boost' dose is indicated, i.e. for inadequate excision, electron beam or implant techniques, delivering a calculated dose of 1,000–1,500 rad, are comparable based on tumor control and sequelae *(Montague, Prosnitz, Ghossein, Clark, Kurtz)*.

Lagios presented evidence that seemingly grossly adequate local excision (segmentectomy) alone is not satisfactory treatment (an arm in an NSABP study). Of 36 patients treated with segmentectomy alone, 9 recurred at the primary site, while none of 7 recurred if radiation therapy was used (average follow-up of 25 months). The frequency of postsegmentectomy local recurrence was higher when carcinoma in-situ was identified at the margins of the specimen than when the margins were clear.

Clark, reporting on 680 patients with 4,000 rad in 16 treatments over 3 weeks at the Princess Margaret Hospital, Toronto, observed that the

Table II. NED survival at 10 years after primary excision plus radiation therapy

Original extent of primary cancer	No further treatm.		Salvage surgery		Total	
	n	%	n	%	n	%
Stage I $(T_{1-2} N_0)$	157/225	70	42/60	70	199/285	70
Stage II $(T_{1-2} N_1)$	94/172	55	37/75	49	131/247	53
Stage III $(T_3 N_{0-1})$	31/80	39	13/44	30	44/124	36

frequency of local failure increased from 7.6% at 5 years to 16.3% at 10 years and then plateaued through 20 years following irradiation.

The marked difference in biological behavior of carcinomas recurring at the primary site in the breast after irradiation compared to chest wall recurrence following total mastectomy of any form was noted by *Kurtz, Clark, Ghossein* and *Prosnitz.*

In a study of 704 patients, with cancers in 'all operable stages' (283 T_1 and T_2 primary cancers were excised while 421 were too large for excision and were biopsied only), *Kurtz* documented that those patients with persistent or locally recurrent primary tumors in the breast, who were treated by mastectomy (79% of the local failures), had the same frequency of survival 10 years later as the entire original group of patients (table II).

Ghossein noted that two-thirds of his patients with local-regional failure were NED 10 years later after salvage surgery. When tumor is found in axillary nodes at the time of salvage surgery, the prognosis is worse (85% NED at 5 years with tumor-free nodes and 50% NED at 5 years with metastases to nodes). Thus, this form of local-regional failure, which is often curable, must be distinguished from postmastectomy chest wall recurrence, usually a biological indicator of incurability.

Survival

Although local-regional tumor control contributes to patient well-being and survival, tumor-free survival is the ultimate objective. Early statistical projections that tumor-free survival for tylectomy plus radiation

Table III. NED survival tylectomy plus radiation therapy

Author	Number of patients	Tumor extent	5 YSR, %	10 YSR, %
Prosnitz	293	stages I and II	72	46
Montague	162	primary <5.0 cm	94 (previous report)	–
Kurtz	225	stage I	–	70
	172	stage II	–	55
Clark	680	stage I (clinical)	83	73
Ghossein	307	T_1	91	–
		T_2	76	–

therapy would equal that following radical mastectomy, are now being substantiated by actual observations (table III).

Sequelae of Treatment

Inasmuch as breast preservation is the primary advantage of conservation surgery plus irradiation, the long-term postirradiation condition of the breast is a major issue. If the preserved breast was not comfortable, functional and cosmetically acceptable to most patients, this form of treatment would be without advocates. Any estimate of cosmesis is highly subjective (table IV).

Many of the reported radiation therapy-related complications occurred during the development of current technique. For example, rib fractures in 11 patients in the study reported by *Prosnitz* have been eliminated by reducing the daily dose to 200 rad or less. Table IV in the paper by *Montague* et al. is representative of the morbidity following meticulous radiation therapy technique.

A long-term risk of major concern is a potential for radiation-induced carcinoma in the breast or other tissue. This risk, although real, often is emphasized irrationally in the perspective of immediate, nonremedial

Table IV. Condition of breast tylectomy plus radiation therapy

Author	% of patients judging condition of their breast to be good to excellent
Ghossein	98
Montague	75

death related to the surgery or anesthetic. Cancer appearing in the treated breast cannot be distinguished from persistence/recurrence of the initial tumor. The risk of developing cancer in the second breast is increased over that of the general population, even without exposure to ionizing radiations.

In a scholarly review, *Levitt* concludes that although 'Caution must be taken because many of the studies were only recently completed and breast cancer following irradiation usually develops after a five to ten year interval, ... there is not an apparent increased risk of second primary breast cancer from irradiation of the first primary breast cancer based on the currently available data.'

Selection of Patients

Much of the initial patient selection in the USA now results from a media-generated awareness of alternatives to mastectomy. *Sacks* noted that about 30% of all patients in his region select an alternative to radical mastectomy.

All females are not candidates for conservation surgery plus radiation therapy. There must be a favorable tumor size-breast size ratio so that tumor excision itself is not deforming. As emphasized by *Westdahl*, a surgeon, and *Montague,* a radiation oncologist, patients who are candidates for this form of treatment must be seen by a surgeon and a radiation oncologist before commitment to treatment. Although criteria of selection varies slightly in different medical centers, *Montague* states that those patients with: large (>4.0 cm) tumors and/or small breasts; very large, pendulous breasts; large of fixed axillary nodes; subareolar primary tumors; or tumors at multiple sites in the breast, usually are not accepted for conservation surgery plus irradiation. *Westdahl* considers that only 25% of the patients he sees are good candidates.

Follow-Up Program

Patients treated by conservation surgery plus radiation therapy have all the usual risks of tumor dissemination plus the potential of persistent or recurrent cancer at the primary site in the breast. An essential aid to evaluation of the irradiated breast is mammography. Noncancer-related, posttreatment changes, i.e. skin thickening and dysplastic calcification, need to be identified *(Montague)*.

Impact of an Alternative to Radical Mastectomy

Effective treatment with conservation of a comfortable, cosmetically acceptable breast should encourage females to seek treatment without fear of disfigurement. *Kelly* noted that fears of disfigurement, death and disruption of life interfere with a female's assessment of personal risk and may be the basis of avoidance of periodic self-examination and visits to a physician.

Vaeth dramatically told of her recent personal experience in selecting an alternative to radical mastectomy in a large US medical center. Her motives were questioned by surgeons, medical oncologists and acquaintances.

A most regrettable impact has been the generation of state legislation with a purported objective of insuring that each patient be made aware of and understands alternative treatments. In the California Health and Safety Code, Section 1704.5, concern is with a single disease, breast cancer. The irony is that apparent reluctance of a surgeon to discuss treatment with a single patient has resulted in a legislative attempt to insure that physicians behave as they should on their own initiative. So far the requirement is that each physician distribute a state-authorized booklet, not yet in existence 7 months following the activation of the law, or face professional discipline. Some differences between legislative attempts in California and Massachusetts have been summarized by *Weinberg* (table V). Such legislative intrusions into medicine are vulnerable to misapplication and raise more questions than they answer. Why not other cancers and other diseases? What about inaccuracies in the booklet?

Based on information presented in this symposium and elsewhere, there is far more documentation that establishes conservation surgery followed by irradiation as a legitimate alternative to mastectomy than

Table V. Comparison of 'Patient's Rights' Legislation in California and Massachusetts

Item	California	Massachusetts
Signed as law	1980 session	May 1979
Effective date	1/1/81	8/21/79
Functioning	–	immediately
Agent	physician	physician
Site of jurisdiction	anywhere	health care facility
Penalties	professional discipline	civil
Informed consent	additional	included

required for many, if not most, therapies enthusiastically endorsed by today's physicians. It now should be a matter of physician education, not legislation. A leading force in this slow educational process is the person most involved: the informed patient.

R.G.Parker, MD, Professor of Radiation Therapy, University of California, Los Angeles, CA (USA)